SALIVARY GLANDS - NEW APPROACHES IN DIAGNOSTICS AND TREATMENT

Edited by **Işıl Adadan Güvenç**

Salivary Glands - New Approaches in Diagnostics and Treatment
http://dx.doi.org/10.5772/intechopen.68846
Edited by Işıl Adadan Güvenç

Contributors

Iordanis Konstantinidis, Angelos Chatziavramidis, Hisao Hiraba, Michihiro Nakayama, Atsutaka Okizaki, Kaori Nakajima, Koji Takahashi, Alejandro Escobar, Juan Pablo Aitken, Goran Mitulović, Karolina Kaczor-Urbanowicz, Anahita Punj, Işıl Adadan Güvenç

Notice

First published in London, United Kingdom, 2019 by IntechOpen
IntechOpen is the global imprint of INTECHOPEN LIMITED, registered in England and Wales, registration number: 11086078, The Shard, 25th floor, 32 London Bridge Street
London, SE19SG – United Kingdom
Printed in Croatia

British Library Cataloguing-in-Publication Data
A catalogue record for this book is available from the British Library

Additional hard copies can be obtained from orders@intechopen.com

Salivary Glands - New Approaches in Diagnostics and Treatment, Edited by Işıl Adadan Güvenç
p. cm.
Print ISBN 978-1-78984-988-2
Online ISBN 978-1-78984-989-9

For EU product safety concerns:
IN TECH d.o.o., Prolaz Marije Krucifikse Kozulić 3, 51000 Rijeka, Croatia,
info@intechopen.com or visit our website at intechopen.com.

Meet the editor

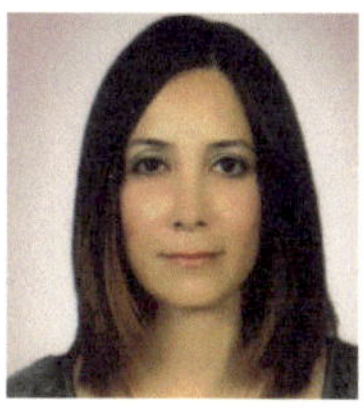

Dr. Işıl Adadan Güvenç was born in 1976 in İzmir, Turkey. After graduating from the American Collegiate Institute in İzmir, she received her medical degree at Hacettepe University, Faculty of Medicine, in 2000. She then specialized in otorhinolaryngology head and neck surgery at İzmir Atatürk Research and Training Hospital. Today, she works in Çiğli Regional Training Hospital in İzmir as an associate professor in ENT. She is a fellow of the European Board of ORL-HNS, and has published 15 articles in respectable international journals and 11 articles in national journals. She is married to an architect and has an 8-year-old son.

Contents

Preface

Saliva is a complex fluid that maintains oral health and possesses important functions in lubrication, digestion, taste perception and speech. Moreover, saliva is a potential noninvasive diagnostic fluid, which provides valuable diagnostic information for detecting numerous diseases. Thanks to the advances in diagnostic methods, the number of studies using salivary analysis in the diagnosis of various diseases and conditions has increased tremendously. As evidence from recent research accumulates, salivary diagnostics will become more easily accepted by clinicians and patients.

Salivary Glands - New Approaches in Diagnostics and Treatment is a comprehensive reference, which brings together information on salivary secretion and its disorders, as well as novel diagnostic methods for numerous diseases with the use of salivary secretions, and new techniques in the treatment of salivary diseases. Therefore, this book contains a source of information for a diverse audience, such as researchers of basic science and clinicians of surgical and medical sciences, including dentists, oral biologists, experimental biologists, molecular biologists, oncologists, radiologists, oral and maxillofacial surgeons, and otorhinolaryngologists.

In the first three chapters of the book, a basic understanding of salivary secretion is provided along with a description and management of conditions that decrease or increase the amount of saliva. The next section of the book introduces the reader to salivary diagnostics, a new diagnostic approach that has the potential to reach clinical practice in the near future for the early detection, diagnosis, and monitoring of many diseases, such as cancer, human papillomavirus infections, dental problems, diabetes, heart diseases, Sjögren's syndrome, and even neurological and psychiatric disorders. Afterwards, the proteomics of saliva are described in detail. Next, scintigraphic techniques for the functional diagnosis of salivary diseases and for distinguishing salivary tumors are discussed. The last two chapters describe a combined endoscopic procedure used in recent years in the treatment of sialolithiasis and a novel method, facial vibrotactile stimulation, for the increase of salivation.

I would like to sincerely thank my husband Erkan Güvenç for his patience, my mother Emel Adadan who was always beside me whenever she was needed, and our nanny Ellie Mikrut who took great care of my dearest Kaan for sacrificing their time and supporting me in making this book happen.

Işıl Adadan Güvenç, MD
Cigli Regional Education Hospital
Izmir, Turkey

Section 1

Salivary Glands and its Diseases

Chapter 1

Secretions of Human Salivary Gland

Anahita Punj

Additional information is available at the end of the chapter

http://dx.doi.org/10.5772/intechopen.75538

Abstract

The salivary glands play an important role in our body by the virtue of its ability to secrete saliva. Saliva has a role to play in maintaining the health of the oral cavity and for carrying out physiological functions like mastication, taste perception, speech etc. It also acts as a mirror to the systemic status of an individual owing to its ability to act as a diagnostic fluid for detecting a number of conditions and diseases. Saliva is a potential non-invasive diagnostic fluid for detection of a number of biomarkers of disease and health. Advancement in diagnostic methods has helped in identifying biomarkers of disease in saliva. In order to understand and diagnose pathological changes, a thorough understanding of the salivary gland anatomy, physiology and regulation of its secretion is warranted. This chapter aims to provide the basic understanding of the secretions of saliva.

Keywords: saliva, secretion, salivary gland, diagnostic fluid

1. Introduction

Salivary glands are organs which synthesize and secrete their secretions over an epithelial surface via a hollow channel. These glands are present in and around the oral cavity and its secretions play an important role in the physiological processes of the oral cavity [1].

2. Overview of salivary glands

The salivary glands can be classified as major and minor salivary glands. The major salivary glands, located outside the oral cavity include the parotid salivary gland, submandibular/submaxillary salivary gland and sublingual salivary gland. The minor salivary glands are classified based on their location in the oral cavity as labial/buccal glands, glossopalatine glands, palatine glands, lingual glands which are further classified as anterior lingual (glands of Blandin and Nuhn) and posterior lingual glands (Von Ebner's) [1, 2]. The following diagram (**Figure 1**) shows the anatomical location of major and minor salivary glands. The salivary glands consists of a secretory part and ducts (**Table 1**).

2.1. Parenchymal elements of salivary gland

The salivary glands are made of secretory units called acini, which are made up of acinar cells which could be serous or mucous. The serous cells are pyramidal or triangular in shape while the mucous cells are columnar in shape. The serous cells are occasionally seen capped by structures called demilunes. The acini cells are surrounded by contractile cells called as myoepithelial cells/basket cells, which are responsible for the flow of secretions of saliva by contraction of the cell. The acini of salivary glands are connected to hollow tubular structures which are called salivary ducts. The lining of the duct changes with the type of duct and its location within the salivary gland [1–3]. A description of the ducts observed is given in **Table 2** and the parenchymal elements are shown in **Figure 2**.

2.2. Development of salivary gland

Salivary glands arise from the ectoderm of oral cavity. The minor salivary gland arise from the oral and nasopharyngeal ectoderm. The chronology of the development of salivary gland is mentioned in **Table 3**. Each gland develops at a specific location in the oral cavity by the inward growth of an epithelial bud into the underlying mesenchyme. These epithelial buds then grow and later branch into a system of cords of cells. These get canalized and develop

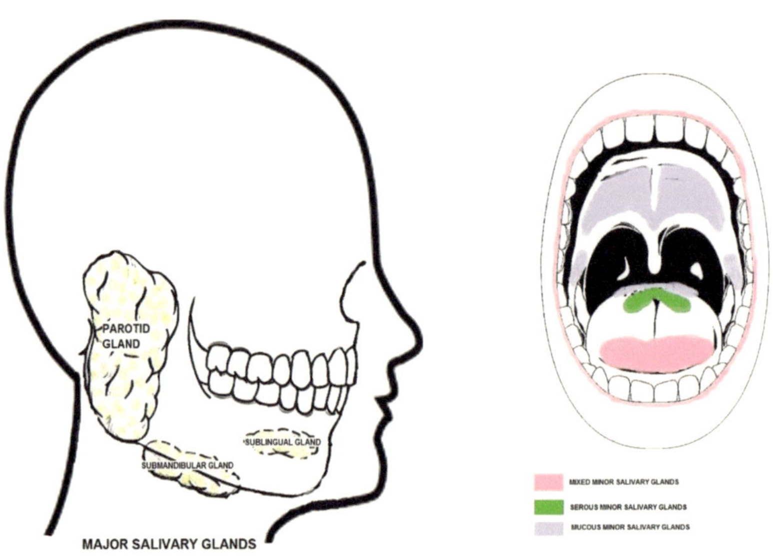

Figure 1. Anatomical locations of major and minor salivary glands.

S. no	Salivary gland	Salivary gland duct	Location of salivary duct orifice
1.	Parotid	Stensen's duct	Opens at papilla in buccal mucosa opposite maxillary second molar
2.	Submandibular	Wharton's duct	Opens at sublingual papillae
3.	Sublingual	Bartholin's duct	Opens with or near submandibular duct
		Duct of Rivinus	Opens independently along sublingual fold
4.	Minor salivary glands	Short ducts	Open directly via short ducts into mouth

Table 1. Location and names of salivary gland ducts.

S. no	Duct	Description	Epithelium
1.	Intercalated duct	Connect the terminal secretory unit with the next system of ducts	Single layer of low cuboidal cells
2.	Striated duct	Intercalated ducts drain into striated duct	Tall columnar epithelial cells with centrally placed nucleus. Cells are partitioned by deep sheet like foldings of membrane, which appear as striations under light microscope
3.	Interlobular duct/ excretory duct	Formed by joining of striated ducts	Pseudo-stratified columnar epithelial cells with outer connective tissue adventitia

Table 2. Description of salivary ducts.

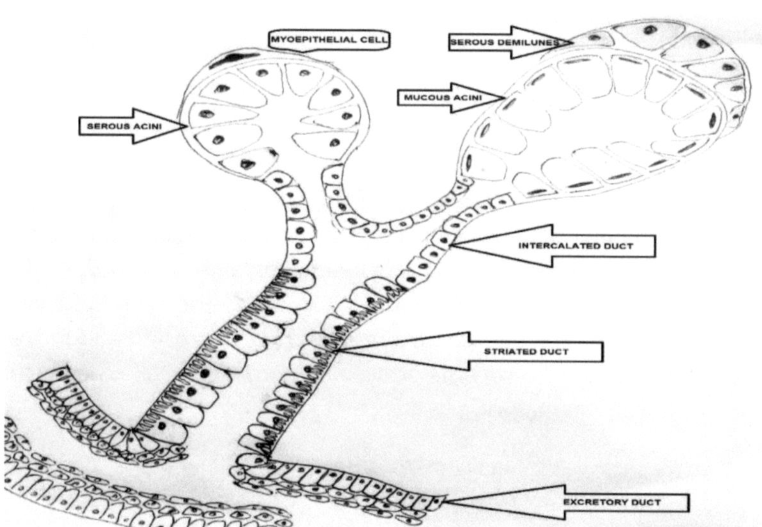

Figure 2. Architecture of salivary ducts and acini.

S. no	Time	Event
1.	Sixth week	Development of the primordia of parotid and submandibular salivary gland
2.	Seventh to eighth week	Development of sublingual salivary gland
3.	Third month	Development of minor salivary gland

Table 3. Chronology of salivary gland development.

a lumen by the action of microfilaments at apical areas of cell to become ducts. The secretory part develops later by repeated branching and budding of finer cell cords, to form pregland cells which give rise to acini [1].

3. Secretions of salivary gland

The salivary glands are primarily involved in secretion of saliva. There are other substances also which are secreted by the salivary glands which are found in saliva. They can secrete proteins in large amounts apically or basolaterally to the saliva [1–4].

3.1. Saliva

Saliva is a complex physiological fluid of the oral cavity which coats the teeth and oral mucosa. It contains a myriad of components like enzymes, mucinous substances, antibacterial components etc. Saliva functions to maintain the oral cavity in the physiological state owing to its lubricating, buffering, antibacterial and immune properties by acting as a physiological barrier to infections. The saliva is a mixed fluid, as it is composed of saliva secreted by both major and minor salivary glands which are both serous and mucous in nature [2–4].

3.1.1. Composition of saliva

Saliva is composed of 99% water and 1% of components such as inorganic ions like sodium, potassium, chloride, bicarbonate, calcium, magnesium, fluoride, thiocyanate, hydrogen phosphate etc. It contains proline-rich proteins, histatins, cystatin, defensins. Kallikrein, cathelicidin-LL37, lactoferrin and enzymes such as amylase (ptyalin), peroxidase, lysozyme, etc. Immunoglobulins A, G and M, glucose, amino acids, urea, uric acid, lipid molecules and blood group antigens, epidermal growth factors, factor VII, factor VIII and factor IX are also present. Saliva in the mouth also consists of desquamated epithelial cells, microorganisms and their products, few inflammatory cells etc. [2–4].

3.1.2. Formation of saliva

According to Tencate [2], the formation of saliva occurs in two stages. The first stage involves the formation of saliva by the acinar cells. The acinar cells whether serous or mucous cells produce salivary secretion by ribosomal protein synthesis in the rough endoplasmic reticulum which is followed by the packaging of the proteins by the golgi complex. The secretions are stored as granules and later released into the lumen by the process of exocytosis or by vesicular mechanism. Exocytosis involves fusion of the secretory granules with the membrane allowing release of the contents into the lumen. Vesicular mechanism involves transport of vesicles filled with secretions from golgi complex to plasma membrane. Transcytosis involves passage of substances like immunoglobulin A through the acini. Water is taken up by the cells from the bloodstream and the resulting saliva secreted is isotonic. The serous cells produce serous saliva which is thin, watery and is composed of zymogen granules and contains more proteins, while mucous cells produce thick, viscous saliva containing mucopolysaccharides and mucin. Parotid gland and von Ebner's gland is purely serous gland, while sublingual, glossopalatine and palatine glands have more of mucous secretions. Submandibular gland and other minor salivary gland have both serous and mucous acini, resulting in mixed saliva [2–6].

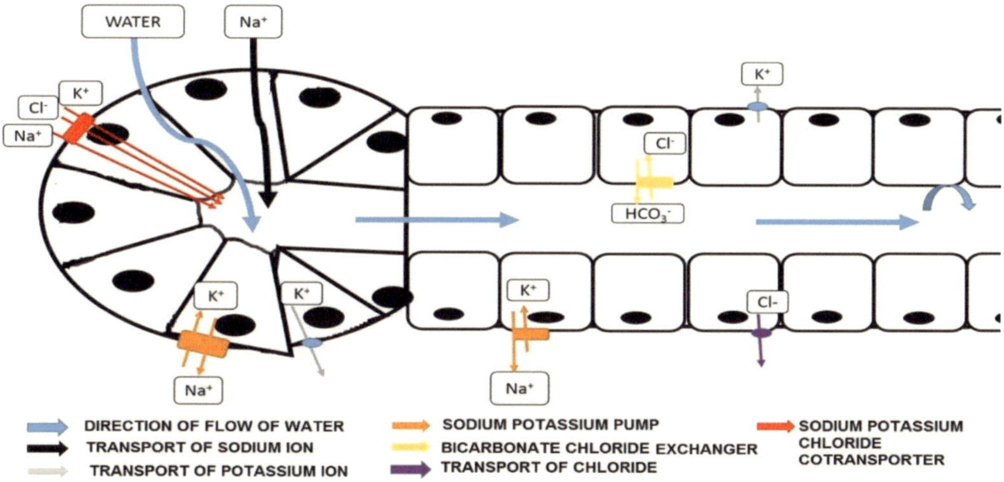

Figure 3. Modification of saliva.

In the second stage the saliva undergoes changes as it passes through the salivary ductal system into the oral cavity. Saliva secreted from the acini is isotonic or slightly hypertonic when it reaches the intercalated ducts. The intercalated duct cells also release lysozymes and lactoferrin. Striated and excretory ducts are impermeable to water. In the striated duct, reabsorption of sodium and chloride occurs more as compared to the secretion of potassium and bicarbonate ions, which makes saliva hypotonic (**Figure 3**). Striated duct cells also secrete kallikrein and epidermal growth factor. Thus, saliva secreted into the oral cavity is hypotonic as compared to serum [1–6].

3.1.3. Saliva secretion in health and disease

The myoepithelial cells are responsible for the contraction of the acini cells, aiding in the flow and secretion of saliva. In health, the total volume of saliva produced is 750–1000 ml daily which is contributed by major and minor salivary glands. The resting flow of saliva is 0.2–0.4 ml/min. Salivary flow at rest refers to as unstimulated saliva, whereas salivary flow in response to a stimulus refers to stimulated saliva having a flow rate of 2–5 ml/min. The normal pH of saliva is 6.4–7.4 [1, 2].

A number of factors control the quality and quantity of saliva secreted. The control of salivary gland secretion is mediated by the autonomic nervous system (ANS). All the salivary gland cells receive ANS supply. Control of secretion is also dependent on the perception of taste and smell. The gustatory stimulus is more important than the masticatory stimulus in controlling the salivary secretion. The secretion of saliva occurs by the process of stimulus secretion coupling. This refers to the events involving release of neurotransmitter from vesicles in nerve terminals adjacent to parenchymal cells which stimulate them to discharge secretory granules, water and electrolytes as well as contraction of myoepithelial cells. Norepinephrine activates both alpha and beta adrenergic receptors, while parasympathetic transmitter like acetylcholine activate cholinergic receptors. Alpha adrenergic receptor stimulation results in protein secretion while beta adrenergic or cholinergic stimulation results in low protein secretion and secretion of water and electrolytes. Substance P stimulates alpha adrenergic and cholinergic secretion of saliva. The following flow chart (**Figure 4**) shows the events associated with stimulus secretion coupling which involves the basic process of receptor stimulation which results in increase in the concentration of a secondary messenger, which will further trigger additional events leading to a cellular response [3–6].

Copious watery saliva is secreted in response to parasympathetic stimulation and thicker saliva in response to sympathetic stimulation. Other factors affecting saliva composition are flow rate, circadian rhythm, duration of stimulus, nature of stimulus and diet. During sleep very little saliva is secreted by major salivary glands and majority of the saliva secreted is by the minor salivary glands. Concentration of saliva depends on rate of flow and not on nature of stimulus [2–6].

Historically, it was suggested that parotid salivary gland secretes a hormone called parotin which was considered to have a protein-anabolic function and deficiency resulted in diseases such as chondrodystrophia fetalis, Kaschin-Beck disease, etc. [7].

An increase in the flow of saliva is referred to as sialorrhea (ptyalism), while a decrease in the salivary flow is referred to as xerostomia (dry mouth). Ptyalism is observed after insertion of new orthodontic appliance, in pregnancy, epilepsy, cerebral palsy and Parkinson's disease. Xerostomia is observed in menopause, patients treated by radiation therapy, old age, prolonged use of tranquilizers, amphetamines, antihypertensive and anticonvulsant drugs. A number of systemic conditions affect the functioning of the secretion of salivary glands. Hyperthyroidism, pernicious anemia, vitamin D deficiency, multiple sclerosis and poorly controlled diabetes mellitus affect the salivary glands. Autoimmune diseases like Sjogren's syndrome, Mikulicz's disease affect the salivary gland secretion as the parenchymal elements are affected. Inflammatory, infective and neoplastic diseases also disrupt the activity of salivary gland secretion. Salivary secretion is influenced by hormones. For example antidiuretic hormone facilitates water reabsorption by striated duct, aldosterone causes increased sodium reabsorption by striated duct, testosterone and thyroxine increase salivary secretion [2, 8, 9].

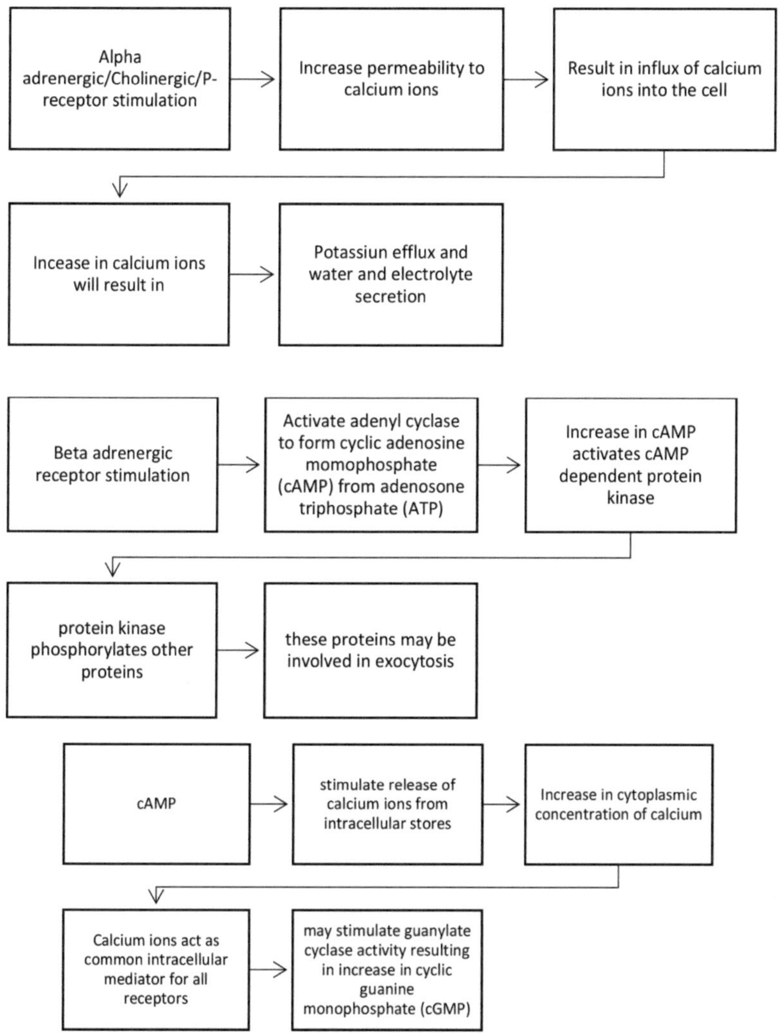

Figure 4. Flowchart depicting sequence of events following neural stimulation.

4. Significance of salivary secretion

The saliva has a number of important functions as mentioned below.

Protection: the saliva contains mucin and glycoproteins which provides it with lubricating properties and moistening the oral cavity, thus preventing friction between the oral structures during physiological functions like mastication. The constant flow of saliva provides clearance of accumulated food debris and microorganisms. Mucins also provide thermal and chemical insulation. Proteins, glycoproteins and mucins form a coating called pellicle formation. Saliva acts as a source of calcium, phosphate, fluoride, statherin and proline rich protein which maintain the integrity of enamel and repair.

Digestion: water and mucin content of saliva aids in bolus formation during the process of mastication. Saliva contains salivary amylase (ptyalin) which helps in digestion of starch and lingual lipase secreted by von Ebner's gland breaks down triglycerides.

Antimicrobial activity: mucins aid in providing a physical barrier to infections by preventing attachment of microorganisms to tooth and tissue surface. Presence of secretory immunoglobulin A provides immune defense. Peroxidase, lysozyme, lactoferrin, histatin, mucins, agglutinin, defensins and cathelicidin also help in providing antimicrobial activity.

Buffering: bicarbonate, phosphate, basic proteins, urea and ammonia help maintain the pH and neutralization of acids.

Tissue repair: salivary glands release growth factors, trefoil proteins into saliva which aid is tissue repair and regeneration.

Taste: saliva acts as a solvent in which molecules from food items can dissolve and reach the taste buds, epidermal growth factor and carbonic anhydrase VI maintains taste buds.

Role of saliva in periodontal pathology: saliva exerts a major influence on plaque initiation, maturation and metabolism. The first step in plaque formation is formation of pellicle followed by plaque formation and maturation [1–6, 8, 9].

Salivary proteins may play a role in plaque mineralization. It is indicated that esterase, pyrophosphatase, acid phosphatase and lysozyme may be involved. Persons with heavy calculus, have higher levels of salivary glycoproteins than non-calculus formers [1–6, 8, 9].

Polymorphonuclear neutrophils (PMNs) reach the oral cavity by migrating through the lining of gingival sulcus. Skougaard and Bay, 1994 believe that orogranulocytic migratory rate correlates with severity of gingival inflammation and is therefore reliable index for assessing gingivitis [8–11].

The saliva acts as an important diagnostic oral fluid owing to its ease and non-invasive mode of collection. A number of components secreted in saliva can be assessed and used to assess diseased states.

A few of the components used as specific biomarkers for detection of periodontal disease include immunoglobulins (Ig) such as IgA, IgM, IgG which interfere in adherence and bacterial metabolism and are present in increased concentration in saliva of chronic and aggressive periodontal patients. Nonspecific markers for aggressive periodontitis include mucins which interfere with the colonization of Aggregatibacter actinomycetemcomitans (A. a), lactoferrin which inhibits microbial growth/increased correlation with A. a. Markers for chronic periodontitis include lysozyme which regulates biofilm accumulation and peroxidase which interferes with biofilm accumulation. Nonspecific markers for both chronic and aggressive periodontitis include histatin which neutralizes lipopolysaccharide and enzymes known to affect periodontium and C-reactive proteins which are present in increased concentrations in saliva and serum of patients with periodontitis [8].

Other areas where saliva can be used for diagnosis of diseases and conditions include cystic fibrosis, which is a genetically transmitted disease of children and young adults characterized by generalized exocrinopathy. In this condition, saliva contains increased calcium levels, elevated levels of sodium and a decrease in flow rate [8, 9].

Sjogren's Syndrome is associated with reduction in lacrimal and salivary secretions. It is characterized by the presence of a lymphocytic infiltrate (predominantly CD4+ T-cells) in the salivary gland parenchyma. A low resting flow rate and abnormally low stimulated flow rate of whole saliva. An antibody p53 can also be detected in the saliva of patients diagnosed with oral squamous cell carcinoma (SCC). Viral diseases like measles, mumps, and rubella can be detected, polymerase chain reaction (PCR)-based identification of virus in saliva is a useful method for the early detection of HSV-1 reactivation in patients with Bell's palsy. Acute hepatitis A (HAV) and hepatitis B (HBV) can be diagnosed based on the presence of Immunoglobulin M antibodies in saliva [8, 9].

Saliva can be used for monitoring of anti-epileptic drugs as a positive correlation between salivary and serum carbamazepine levels has been observed. In another study, salivary levels of phenobarbital and phenytoin demonstrated excellent correlations with serum levels of these medications. Other drugs that can be identified in saliva are amphetamines, barbiturates, benzodiazepines, cocaine, phencyclidine (PCP), and opioids [8–10].

Steroid hormones can be detected in saliva. Salivary cortisol levels were found to be useful in identifying patients with Cushing's syndrome and Addison's disease [12].

Recent focus on the potential role of periodontal disease as a risk factor for cardiovascular and cerebrovascular diseases [13, 14] and the occurrence of pre-term low-birth-weight babies [15] bring new importance to this aspect of salivary analysis [8–15].

Salivary markers as potential diagnostic tests for periodontal disease include proteins of host origin (i.e., enzymes, immunoglobulins), phenotypic markers, host cells, hormones (cortisol), bacteria and bacterial products, ions and volatile compounds [8, 9, 11].

Salivary levels of MMP-8 and IL-1β appear to serve as biomarkers of alveolar bone loss and hence periodontitis [8, 9, 11].

National Institute of Dental and Craniofacial Research, has highlighted the use of saliva for translational and clinical application by use of salivary proteome and the salivary transcriptome for early detection, disease progression and therapeutic monitoring [8, 9].

Gene therapy has been developed to deliver growth hormone in deficiency states by salivary gland expression of growth hormone [16].

5. Conclusion

The secretions of salivary gland form an integral part of maintaining the physiology of the oral cavity. Saliva is the most important and essential secretion of the salivary glands. Saliva itself has varied functions in the oral cavity and provides additional insight and details of the systemic status of the individual as well. With the advancement in the field of proteomics, transcriptomics and genomics, better and easier methods of detecting diseases by analyzing saliva are being discovered. For this reason the study of salivary glands and its secretion becomes needful.

Conflict of interest

There is no conflict of interest.

Author details

Anahita Punj

Address all correspondence to: anahitapunj@gmail.com

Army College of Dental Sciences, Secunderabad, Telangana, India

References

[1] Kumar GS. Orban's Oral Histology & Embryology. 13th ed. India: Reed Elsevier India Private Limited; 2011

[2] Nanci A. Salivary Glands. TenCate's Oral Histology Development, Structure and Function. 8th ed. South Asia edition. India: Reed Elsevier India Private Limited; 2012. pp. 253-277

[3] Proctor GB. The physiology of salivary secretion. Periodontology 2000. 2016;**70**:11-25

[4] Tiwari M. Science behind human saliva. Journal of Natural Science, Biology, and Medicine. 2011;**2**(1):53-58. DOI: 10.4103/0976-9668.82322

[5] Lavelle CLB. Saliva. Applied Oral Physiology. 2nd ed. London, Boston, Singapore, Sydney, Toronto, Wellington: Wright; 1988. pp. 128-141

[6] Bradley RM. Salivary Secretion. Essentials of Oral Physiology. Missouri: Mosby; 1995. pp. 161-185

[7] Ito Y. Parotin: A salivary gland hormone. Annals of the New York Academy of Sciences. 1960;**85**:228-312. DOI: 10.1111/j.1749-6632.1960.tb49961.x

[8] Giannobile WV, Beikler T, Kinney JS, Ramseier CA, Morelli T, Wong DT. Saliva as a diagnostic tool for periodontal disease: Current state and future directions. Periodontology 2000. 2009;**50**:52-64. DOI: 10.1111/j.1600-0757.2008.00288.x

[9] Miller CS, King CP Jr, Langub MC, Kryscio RJ, Thomas MV. Salivary biomarkers of existing periodontal disease: A cross-sectional study. Journal of the American Dental Association. 2006;**137**(3):322-329

[10] Skougaard MR, Bay I, Klinkhamer JM. Correlation between gingivitis and orogranulocytic migratory rate. Journal of Dental Research. 1969;**48**(5):716-718

[11] Newman MG, Klokkevold PR, Takei HH, Carranza FA. Carranza's Clinical Periodontology. 10th ed. Philadelphia: Saunders; 2009

[12] Hubl W, Taubert H, Freymann E, Meissner D, Stahl F, Dorner G. A sensitive direct enzyme immunoassay for cortisol in plasma and saliva. Experimental and Clinical Endocrinology. 1984;**84**:63-70

[13] Joshipura KJ, Douglass CW, Willett WC. Possible explanations for the tooth loss and cardiovascular disease relationship. Annals of Periodontology. 1998;**3**(1):175-183

[14] Morrison HI, Ellison LF, Taylor GW. Periodontal disease and risk of fatal coronary heart and cerebrovascular diseases. Journal of Cardiovascular Risk. 1999;**6**(1):7-11

[15] Offenbacher S, Beck JD, Lieff S, Slade G. Role of periodontitis in systemic health: Spontaneous preterm birth. Journal of Dental Education. 1998;**62**(10):852-858

[16] Racz GZ, Zheng C, Goldsmith CM, Baum BJ, Cawley NX. Towards gene therapy for growth hormone deficiency via salivary gland expression of growth hormone. Oral Diseases. 2015;**21**(2):149-155. DOI: 10.1111/odi.12217

Chapter 2

Xerostomia: An Update of Causes and Treatments

Alejandro Escobar and Juan P. Aitken-Saavedra

Additional information is available at the end of the chapter

http://dx.doi.org/10.5772/intechopen.72307

Abstract

Xerostomia or dry mouth sensation is considered a complex condition that affects several stomatological functions that drives to the detriment of the quality of life of individuals who suffer from it. Often, xerostomia is accompanied by a decrease in salivary flow or hyposalivation, and this condition leads to oral health problems such as dental caries, candidiasis, and mucosal complications. Currently, the diagnosis and therapeutic methods for this condition are varied and it is difficult to achieve favorable results in all cases, since the etiology seems to be multifactorial where both local factors and systemic conditions would participate. This chapter presents, in a concise shape, the relevant data about etiology of xerostomia, such as age, autoimmune diseases, systemic diseases, infectious diseases, neuropathic complications, psychogenic factors and therapeutically consumption of drugs among others, and the current available treatments.

Keywords: xerostomia, etiology, diagnosis, clinical manifestation, treatments

1. Introduction

Xerostomia or dry mouth sensation is considered a complex condition that affects several stomatological functions and drives to the detriment of the quality of life of individuals who suffer from it. Often, xerostomia is accompanied by a decrease in salivary flow or hyposalivation with consequences such as oral lesions, alterations of taste, feeling of thick saliva, chewing problems, dental caries, dental demineralization, periodontal disease, salivary gland infection, cervical caries, fungal infections, and others [1]. Currently, the diagnosis and therapeutic methods for this condition are varied and it is difficult to achieve favorable results in all cases, since the etiology seems to be multifactorial where both local and systemic factors would participate [2–5]. Although xerostomia may occur frequently in the general population, clear and defined tools for diagnosis and treatment are still needed. Today, patients suffering from xerostomia visit numerous health professionals to solve this complex condition that limits many functions of day-to-day life, and often does not find response or effective treatment. Regards the complexity of xerostomia and its importance in dental practice, this chapter reviews the relevant data about etiology, diagnosis, consequences, and the current available treatments to this condition.

2. Definition and evaluation

Xerostomia (dry mouth, oral dryness, and mouth dryness) is the dryness of oral cavity and can be caused by lower salivary flow or the complete lack of saliva [6]. Based on the etiology, the xerostomia can be classified as true xerostomia (xerostomia vera, primaria), caused by the malfunction of the salivary glands and pseudo xerostomia or symptomatic xerostomia (xerostomia spuria, symptomatica), which is described as the subjective sensation of oral dryness, despite normal secretory function of the salivary glands [7]. The xerostomia, as a symptom, is more common in older populations, but its causes are not related to aging. It has been shown it is related to some specific diseases, drugs, or therapies associated [8]. The prevalence of xerostomia varies from 13 to 28% in older populations, and increases up to 60% in patients living in long-term care facilities [9–11].

Xerostomia, although not considered a disease, may imply the presence of changes directly related to the salivary glands or be the result of systemic diseases [12]. In order for a suitable treatment to be instituted in a timely manner, it is important to carry out a thorough evaluation of the patient with the dry mouth condition, determining, if possible, the cause of the xerostomia. The patients with xerostomia, who are present with salivary gland hypofunction, are at risk of many oral complications; the persistence over time of low rates of salivary secretion causes changes in the oral environment and affects the hard and soft tissues of the mouth. Xerostomia can also be a consequence of systemic disease and its recognition is a valuable aid in the treatment [13]. It is a potentially debilitating condition that can affect up to 1 in 5 oncology patients, with higher prevalence in women and the elderly. There is evidence that the use of multiple medications may increase the risk of xerostomia [13]. This symptom represents a strong impact on the quality of life of the people affected. Over 87.6% of people with xerostomia were worried if they had to spend the rest of their lives with the dry mouth sensation [14]. The dry mouth (xerostomia) sensation has a higher incidence on individuals over 60 years old (12–40%), up to three times higher than on younger adults. It does not seem to be directly related to the normal aging process, but to some chronic diseases or treatments [15, 16]. It is estimated that about 20–30% of the 20-year-old population has xerostomia and the cause may be the increased use of antidepressants, since xerostomia is associated with depression and anxiety. In United States, up to 40% of the 20-year-old population may have xerostomia. The high consumption of antidepressants and other medications, as well as alcoholic beverages and tobacco may explain the increase in people with this condition [17].

Although xerostomia, as a symptom, entails many problems for patients who suffer from it, especially in relation to their quality of life, the decrease in the amount of saliva due to its multiple properties is what brings more consequences at the oral level. Saliva is composed of 99% water and electrolytes. The rest of the composition is organic and includes immunoglobulins, digestive enzymes such as amylase and lipase, and antibacterial and antifungal enzymes, as well as mucins [14]. Ninety-three percent of its volume is secreted by the major salivary glands and the remaining 7% by the minor glands. Saliva production is controlled by the autonomous nervous system, mainly by parasympathetic nerve signals [18]. Saliva is very important for the preservation of general and oral homeostasis. It has a participation in digestives functions, cleaning, sense of taste, oral mucosa hydration, and defense of teeth trough pH control and its remineralizing potential. In addition, it has antimicrobial properties and controls the composition of oral microbiota by its antibacterial, antiviral, and antifungal capacities [14]. A summary of the Saliva components and functions can be seen in **Table 1**.

Several short and long-term conditions can interrupt salivary secretion, leading to xerostomia. Xerostomia can thus result from three basic causes:

(1) Factors affecting the salivary center: psychological problems (stress and anxiety), Parkinson's disease, Alzheimer's disease (changes in the ability to perceive oral sensations), menopause, and others;

(2) Factors that alter nerve stimulation of saliva: encephalitis, brain tumors, smoking and dehydration (resulting from the deficiency of water intake, vomiting, diarrhea and polyuria), as well as the use of some drugs, including antihistamines, opioids, antidepressants, antiepileptics, anxiolytics, anticholinergics, antimuscarinics, and others;

(3) Alterations in salivary gland function as a consequence of obstruction, infection (sialodenitis), glandular tumors, calculi (sialolithiasis), autoimmune diseases (Sjögren's syndrome-SS-, rheumatoid arthritis, uncontrolled diabetes mellitus and systemic lupus erythematosus), and chemotherapy or radiotherapy performed as cancer therapy for the head and neck area. The extent of injury induced by radiotherapy depends on the volume of irradiated glands and the total dose and technique used [15, 19–23].

Functions	**Components**
Digestion	Amylase, lipase, ribonucleases, proteases, water, mucins
Phonation	Water, mucin
Taste	Water, gustin
Lubrication	Mucin, proline-rich glycoproteins, water
Antimicrobial action	Lysozyme, lactoferrin, lactoperoxides, mucins, cystins, histatins, immunoglobulins, proline-rich glycoproteins, IgA
Maintaining mucosa integrity	Mucins, electrolytes, water
Cleansing	Water
Buffer capacity and remineralization	Bicarbonate, phosphate, calcium, staterin, proline-rich anionic proteins, fluoride
Preparing food for swallowing	Water, mucins Digestion Amylase, lipase, ribonucleases, proteases, water, mucins

Table 1. Saliva components and functions.

3. Diagnosis of xerostomia

The objective of the diagnosis is to provide treatment as early as possible, thus minimizing side effects in patients suffering from xerostomia. In order to establish a diagnosis of xerostomia, a clinical history is essential to identify the possible etiological factors [24]. It is necessary to investigate its causes. Thus, three orders of factors need to be known: the occurrence of systemic diseases, medication, and the history of radiation therapy. Questions are asked to the patient, trying to find out if he feels the dry mouth sensation, whether he needs to wet his mouth, if he can eat a wafer without drinking water, if the tongue chews the food and clings to the teeth, and the daily water intake daily among other issues [24, 25]. The qualitative clinical diagnosis of xerostomia is made through the observation of clinical signs such as palpation of the salivary glands, observation of the oral mucosa and its hydration, cracked lips, saliva under the tongue, appearance and texture of saliva, the identification of caries, candidiasis and burning sensation, and others [26].

Several methods have been developed to evaluate the level of dryness of the mouth, the discomfort being the most used: sialography, sialochemistry, sialometry and scintigraphy, salivary gland biopsy, ultrasound, magnetic resonance, and computed tomography [19]. Sialography is a technique of imaging that involves the injection of a retrograde form of radiopaque material into the salivary duct system in order to define the anatomy of the glands. This test is very important to demonstrate the presence of nodules or sialectasis, but it has its disadvantages, such as: the difficulty of the technique, since it is invasive and the patient can react acutely or chronically with the contrast material. The biopsy of the major or minor salivary glands allows the detection of inflammatory infiltrations, acinar destruction and dilation of salivary channels with thick mucus, and sometimes fibrosis [27]. Ultrasound, magnetic resonance, and computed tomography are tests that may also contribute to the diagnosis of diseases of the salivary glands.

To establish the condition of the symptom or to evaluate a possible salivary glandular dysfunction, the most used mechanisms are the questionnaire of xerostomia developed by Fox et al. [11, 28] and the determination of salivary flow rate. Sialometry and scintigraphy (an imaging diagnostic method of nuclear medicine that allows the study of the physiology of the various organs) are complementary tests that must be performed in order to evaluate the involvement of the salivary glands in patients with xerostomia. Sialometry is a relatively common procedure in normal clinical practice and include determination of stimulated salivary flow rate (s-SFR), unstimulated salivary flow rate (u-SFR), palatal secretion (PAL), and parotid secretion (PAR). These measurements are the simplest methods of evaluating the salivary glandular function. It is essential to measure the salivary flow, that is, the amount of saliva produced per unit of time. Very low unstimulated and stimulated salivary flow rates or hyposalivation are defined as <0.1 and <0.7 mL/min, respectively [7]. At rest, secretion ranges from 0.25 to 0.35 mL/min and is mostly produced by the submandibular and sublingual glands [29]. Under stimulation, the parotids account for 50% of salivary volume [30]. Determining the stimulated and unstimulated salivary flow is a procedure to measure the amount of saliva it produces a person at a given time. Generally, the stimulated salivary flow is measured for 5 min and unstimulated salivary flow is measured for 15 min [31]. This kind of measuring has the advantage of being easily implemented, low-cost, and could be available to most of the population at risk [32]. The diagnosis of salivary gland dysfunction is based on data derived from the symptoms reported by the patient, clinical examination leading to verification of the clinical signs and determination of stimulated salivary flow [33]. A severe decrease in salivary flow may lead to a poor health-related quality of life, as well as a risk condition for the development of oral pathologies such as periodontal disease, caries, and candidiasis [29, 34, 35].

4. Causes of xerostomia

The most severe conditions with effect on the salivary flow are SS and radiotherapy in the head and neck area, with the prevalence of xerostomia in almost 100% in these cases. These conditions are characterized by a progressive loss of secretory cells, and thus a progressive decline in saliva production [36, 37]. Less severe conditions may be dehydration, smoking, and inflammation or infection of the salivary glands [12]. In older people, the most common cause of xerostomia is the use of medications because the vast majority of the elderly are being treated with at least one drug that causes salivary hypofunction [32]. A summary of the main causes of xerostomia can be seen in **Table 2**.

4.1. Aging

The reduced salivary flow is commonly seen in the aging populations. This can be attributed to either age-related localized degeneration of salivary glands or systemic diseases [38, 39]. As the patient ages, the organs atrophy and often result in a decrease in salivary production. It was described that in older people the loss was about 30% of acinar cells, with substitution of secretory components by fibrous and adipose tissue [40]. Besides, there are changes in salivary levels of potassium, sodium, IgA, proline-rich protein, lactoferrin, and lysozyme in elderly [28, 40]. A reduction in salivary flow of older people was identified, even in those not using systemic drugs, suggesting a relation between salivary dysfunction and aging [41]. Smith determined that a stimulated salivary flow in healthy adults older than age 70 is lower than in adults under 50 [42].

Systemic diseases	Sjogren's syndrome, diabetes mellitus, Parkinson's disease, encephalitis, brain tumors, Plummer Vinson disease, hypertension, HIV infection, systemic rheumatic diseases, sarcoidosis, Alzheimer's disease, cystic fibrosis, aplasia, chronic tuberculosis, primary biliary cirrhosis, hemolytic anemia, malignant lymphoma, systemic lupus erythematosus, scleroderma, dermatomyositis, pernicious anemia, hypothyroidism, amyloidosis
Other causes of xerostomia (no drugs or systemic diseases)	Radiotherapy and chemotherapy, infections, inflammation, tumors and sialolithiasis in salivary glands, salivary gland excision, vitamin A deficiency, menopause, stress, anxiety, dehydration, neurological disorders, senility, oral sensory dysfunction, iron deficiency, folic acid deficiency, uremia, polyuria, diarrhea, mouth breathing, bone marrow transplantation, endocrine disorders, pancreatic insufficiency

Table 2. Systemic diseases and other causes of xerostomia.

4.2. Drugs

The most common cause of xerostomia is the use of some systemic medications [43]. Several drugs are able to induce hyposalivation and xerostomia, but they rarely cause irreversible damage to the salivary glands. Over 400 medicines, many of them in common use, induce salivary gland hypofunction [44]. Some examples are: anxiolytics, anticonvulsants, antidepressants, antiemetics, antihistamines, antiparkinsonian, antipsychotics, bronchodilators, decongestants, diuretics, muscle relaxants, analgesics, sedatives and anti-hypertensives, and others (**Table 3**) [29]. The exact mechanisms whereby some drugs determine xerostomia or hyposalivation are still unknown. Salivary dysfunction associated to drugs may occur through anticholinergic, cytotoxic action, sympathomimetic, or by damaged ion transport pathways in the acinar cells [39, 45, 46]. Patients who consume a higher number of daily medications have been associated with complaints of xerostomia [47, 48]. The therapeutic and controlled doses of medications do not damage the salivary gland structure. For that reason, drug-induced xerostomia is reversible. The discontinued use of these drugs can restore salivary flow [49].

4.3. Systemic conditions

Xerostomia or hyposalivation may be caused by local factors, including salivary gland disease (sialadenitis) or salivary gland destruction associated with head and neck irradiation for the

Medicine group	Examples
Anxiolytics	Lorazepam, diazepam
Anorectic	Fenfluramine
Anticonvulsants	Gabapentin
Antidepressants—tricyclic	Amitriptyline, imipramine
Antidepressants—SSRI	Sertraline, fluoxetine
Antiemetics	Meclizine
Antihistaminics	Loratadine
Antiparkinsonian	Biperidene, selegiline
Antipsychotics	Clozapine, chlorpromazine
Bronchodilators	Ipratropium, albuterol
Decongestants	Pseudoephedrine
Diuretics	Spironolactone, furosemide
Muscle relaxants	Baclofen
Narcotic analgesics	Meperidine, morphine
Sedatives	Flurazepam
Antihyperptensive	Prazosin hydrochloride
Antiarthritic	Piroxicam

Table 3. Medicines and drugs with side effects on salivary secretion.

http://dx.doi.org/10.5772/intechopen.72307

treatment of cancer [11, 50]. The effects of radiation are dose, time, and field dependent. When the damage of salivary glands by radiation happens is severe [39] permanent gland damage can be expected if the radiation exposure exceeds 50 Gy [50, 51]. Other systemic conditions that also affect the salivary flow are autoimmune diseases (SS, rheumatoid arthritis, AIDS, systemic lupus erythematosis, and scleroderma), neurological disorders (Parkinson's), psychogenic illness such as depression and hormonal disorders (thyroid dysfunction and diabetes mellitus) [9]. Regarding diabetes, we will refer more deeply about it since it is the most frequent metabolic disease in the world and the trend demonstrates that it continues to grow. Both diabetes mellitus (DM) type 1, as type 2 have been associated with xerostomia. In diabetic subjects were shown that salivary flow was significantly lower than in nondiabetic subjects [49]. The causes of low salivary flow may be due to direct injury in the gland parenchyma, changes in the microcirculation to the salivary glands, glycemic control disorders, and dehydration. Some studies consider that this decrease in salivary flow in diabetic subjects is related to an increased diuresis or polyuria, involving a decrease in extracellular fluid and consequently in saliva production [10]. Others explain this as a consequence of dehydration from glycosuria that would be more evident in cases of metabolic decompensation [52]. Regarding neurological diseases, studies have demonstrated that the salivary flow is lower in Parkinson's disease patients. This phenomenon could contribute to dysphagia, which affects up to 75% of patients with this disease [53]. Autonomic dysfunction could explain the decrease in salivary flow in subjects with this disease and the drugs used to their treatment could increase the problem [54]. One of the diseases most associated with a xerostomia is SS, a condition that involves dry mouth and dry eyes and that may be accompanied by rheumatoid arthritis or a related connective tissue disease. The oral manifestations observed in this disease are attributed to the involvement of the salivary glands, which leads to a decrease in salivary secretion [31, 39]. Patients with depression can have hyposalivation medication-induced. However, xerostomia may be of psychological origin. A study observed that subjects with a subjective sensation of dry mouth were significantly more depressive than non-depressive subjects [55]. Another study indicates the possibility of depression as an underlying factor of the sensation of dry mouth [56].

5. Consequences of xerostomia

Patients with xerostomia may have oral and dental consequences. Xerostomia can seriously impact quality of life and may alter speech, eating, and swallowing [13]. The most common complaints of patients with xerostomia include oral discomfort, difficulty speaking, dysphagia, dysgeusia (decreased taste), feeling of thick saliva, and generally, chewing issues, dental caries, dental demineralization, periodontal disease, salivary gland infection (sialodenitis), oral microflora alterations, burning sensation, mucosal inflammation, sore throats, hoarseness, ulcerations, halitosis, mucosal dehydration, reduced lubrication, painful tongue (glossodynia), enlarged parotid gland, oral mucosal fracture, inflammation and fissures of the lips (cheilitis). The reduction of rates of elimination of substances can affect the palate and be associated with changes in the mouth microbiota. The reduction of rates of elimination of substances can affect the palate and be associated with changes in the mouth microbiota. From the mouth, alterations of taste and intolerance to acidic or spicy foods, dry foodstuffs like biscuits can be very uncomfortable for them, and oral cavity examination may exhibit signs such as fissures on the tongue and lips, angular cheilitis, and dry mucosa. Also, caries, candidiasis, halitosis, or loss of appetite and weight could be observed [25, 57, 58]. This collection of clinical parameters has been indicated as simply estimated for recognizing most patients with xerostomia [38, 47].

The side effects associated with xerostomia are microbial colonization and proliferation in the oral cavity, dental or decreased demineralization, accumulation of stones in the teeth, dehydration of the mucosa, reduction of rates of elimination of substances from the mouth and lubrication of the oral mucosa reduced [13]. When the production of saliva decreases, the buffering capacity of the saliva is reduced, and thus the environment of the oral cavity is vulnerable to acidification, which in addition to determining changes in the normal flora (ecological imbalance) has contributed to the increase in the number of some microorganisms such as *Candida albicans* (a salivary flow less than 0.1 mL/min may cause an increase in the incidence of this fungus) and *Streptococcus mutans* (Gram-negative bacteria). A higher proportion of these microorganisms results in greater acidification of the oral cavity environment, and thus contribute to the enamel demineralization and caries progression. There is a study related to it in which subjects with low salivary flow rate also had significantly more dental caries compared to those with a higher saliva flow rate [58]. In addition, high caries prevalence has been reported to be associated with significantly poorer quality of life compared to low caries prevalence [13].

The infection of the oral mucosa with *C. albicans* affects the lubrication of oral tissues, favoring an increase in the risk of caries and severity of periodontal disease. Candidiasis can also cause burning sensation, glossodynia, glossitis, and angular cheilitis (in areas where the lips are dry or cracked). Patients with prostheses may have reduced retention of the prostheses, pain, and ulcers [59]. The prevalence of oral Candida in the normal population has been estimated to range from 23 to 68% and 68 to 100% among SS patients. Studies have attributed the higher prevalence of oral Candida carriage in this disease to xerostomia [60].

6. Treatments

Treatment design to alleviate dry-mouth symptoms should be personalized to the individual patient, based on available treatment. The treatments of xerostomia can be classified into the following categories: (1) patient education, (2) prevention, (3) symptomatic treatment, (4) systemic and topical salivary stimulants, and (5) regenerative and gene therapies.

6.1. Patient education

Patients should receive detailed information about the potential causes of dry mouth and the potential sequelae of impaired salivary secretion, such as dental caries, candidiasis, and mucosal complications. Therefore, patients should be encouraged to have preventive oral health care such as dental hygiene habits and regular dental visits [61]. Another palliative action to minimizing symptoms and preventing oral complications is water intake, drinking water frequently, and remaining hydrated is an important treatment for symptoms of dry mouth [1].

6.2. Preventive therapies

Pharmacological interventions for the prevention of radiation-induced salivary gland dysfunction have been studied. The use of chemical radioprotectors represents an obvious strategy to improve the therapeutic index in radiotherapy. However, the vast majority of these are either too weak in terms of radioprotection, too toxic, or without any apparent mechanisms to ensure selective normal tissue protection [62]. The sulfhydryl compound amifostine (WR-2721; 2-[(3-aminopropyl) amino] ethylphosphorothioic acid), is an oxygen scavenger that may protect salivary glands from free-radical damage during radiation therapy without attenuation of the anti-tumor effects in many experiments performed [63]. Amifostine has been approved for prevention of xerostomia, in head and neck squamous cell carcinoma patients undergoing radiotherapy [64]. A recent systematic review that included randomized controlled trials suggested that the drug amifostine prevents the feeling of dry mouth in people receiving radiotherapy to head and neck (with or without chemotherapy) in the short- (end of radiotherapy) to medium-term (3 months after radiotherapy) [65]. However, amifostine has adverse effects such as nausea, vomiting, hypotension, transient, hypocalcemia, and allergic reactions [66]. Then, the benefits of amifostine should be weighed against its high cost and side effects. Another cytoprotective compound described in literature is the bioactive factor Keratinocyte growth factor-1 (KGF-1, also known as FGF-7) [67]. In a phase II Study, recombinant KGF (Palifermin) appeared to reduce mucositis, dysphagia, and xerostomia during hyperfractionated radiotherapy but not standard radiation therapy [68].

Current preventative therapies also include surgical salivary glands relocation outside the radiation field [69]. Jha et al. described a surgical transfer of a submandibular salivary gland to the submental space in order to prevent radiation-induced xerostomia in patients with neoplasias of the pharynx and larynx [70].

6.3. Symptomatic treatment

Saliva substitutes can provide some relief since provide higher viscosity and protection to the oral mucosa [39]. An ideal saliva substitute must simulate natural human saliva, providing long lasting and intense hydration of the oral mucosa, be inexpensive, edible, easy-to-swallow but retainable in the mouth and should allow a minimal number of applications [71]. Saliva substitutes are available in various formulations, e.g., lozenges, sprays, mouth rinses, gels, oils, chewing gums, or toothpastes. Most available in the market contain carboxymethylcellulose (CMC), mucins, xanthan gum, hydroxyethylcellulose, linseed oil, or polyethylene oxide [72]. Subjective impressions of patients suffering from severe xerostomia showed that artificial saliva containing mucins and xanthan gum are better in their rheological and moisturizing properties than those with CMC [73], because mucin-based substitutes had viscosities that were more similar to natural saliva. Recently, it was reported that a polysaccharide-based oral rinse was effective in symptom control in patients with xerostomia and may lead to an increase in saliva production [74]. Other studies include the use of natural products, in this line, a recent double-blinded, placebo-controlled clinical trial, evaluated the efficacy of topical lycopene-enriched virgin olive oil. It showed an improvement of oral quality of life and reduction of xerostomia symptoms [75]. Also, gelatinous substitutes of saliva showed a significant reduction of the dryness-related complaints in patients suffering from severe xerostomia [76]. A randomized, double-blind, crossover study in patients affected by medication-induced xerostomia showed that two commercial mouthwash plus gel (GUM® Hydral versus Biotène® Oralbalance) achieve a significant improvement in oral health and xerostomia-related quality of life [77]. Recently, a novel edible saliva substitute, oral moisturizing jelly (OMJ), showed a higher grade of satisfaction than a commercially available saliva gel [78]. In addition to the persistent feeling of dry mouth, people who suffer from xerostomia are very susceptible to bacterial, fungal, and other transmittable mouth infections. It is important that products also include human saliva's enzymes (lactoperoxidase, lysozyme, and lactoferrin). Other important feature is to obtain a continuous oral lubrication. In this context, advances in hydrogel technologies and development of buccal mucoadhesive polymers, allows the continuous release of substances that maintain oral hydration and also offer dental-care benefits for its use in treatment of xerostomia [79]. Other strategy involves the use of modified prosthetic structure designed to retain saliva or substitutes in patients who usually wear a dental prosthesis [4, 80].

6.4. Systemic and topical salivary stimulants

Pilocarpine and cevimeline are two systemic US Food and Drug Administration-approved systemic sialogogues for treatment of dry mouth; both can increase secretions and diminish xerostomic complaints in patients, although they must have functional salivary gland cells. Pilocarpine is a cholinergic parasympathomimetic agent that stimulates muscarinic cholinergic receptors on the surfaces of exocrine glands [81] and has been indicated for the treatment of xerostomia [2, 82]. The usual oral dosage for pilocarpine is 5–10 mg three times per day. The initial recommended dose is 5 mg three times per day oral route (OR), which can be increased up to 30 mg/day depending on response and tolerance. The onset of action is 30 min, and the duration of action is approximately 2–3 h. Common side effects include gastrointestinal upset, sweating, tachycardia, bradycardia, increased pulmonary secretions, increased smooth muscle tone, and blurred vision. Contraindications include gall bladder disease, angle closure glaucoma, and renal colic [39, 83]. Cevimeline is a salivary gland stimulant with a stronger affinity for M3 muscarinic receptors [84]. Since it has no effect on M2 receptors, it shows fewer adverse effects when compared to pilocarpine, and besides, it has a long lasting action. The recommended dose is 30 mg three times a day OR, and the most common associated side effect is dyspepsia. Bethanecol is another drug whose action mechanism is on M3 receptors. It has been used to decrease unwanted effects caused by antidepressant and antipsychotic drugs [85]. The dose indicated is four times a day in doses from 10 to 50 mg OR. Adverse effects, despite being infrequent, include nausea and diarrhea. Other drugs that have been put forward include drug with mucolytic properties such us bromhexine improved salivary secretion in patients with SS [86, 87]. Nizatidine, an H2 receptor antagonist alone or in combination with cisapride, showed a significant increase in salivary secretions of dry mouth patients [88, 89]. In addition, other drugs, such as neostigmine, distigmine, yohimbine, nicotinic, and malic acid have also been attributed positive effects in the treatment of xerostomia [3]. Medicinal herbs, such as jaborandi, betel nut, Iceland Moss and Longo Vital, also can stimulate salivary secretion [4].

In the case of tissue autoimmune-related xerostomia, immunologic agents have been used. Interferon alpha (IFN-α), a protein with antiviral and immunomodulating traits, was an effective treatment for xerostomia linked to SS, improved salivary output and decreased complaints of xerostomia without causing significant adverse medical events [7, 90]. Rituximab (anti-CD20 monoclonal antibody) and infliximab (anti-tumoral necrosis factor—TNF—monoclonal antibody) improved subjective and objective symptoms related to primary SS [91].

Topical salivary stimulants includes sugar-free chewing gum and jellybeans, they can increase salivary secretion by mechanical stimulation and improve the sensation of dry mouth. These products usually contain fluoride, chlorhexidine, calcium phosphate, and xylitol releasers [92, 93], which inhibits the growth of cariogenic bacteria and reduces the incidence of caries [94]. Direct stimulation with electrostimulating device mounted on an intra-oral removable appliance has been used in patients with salivary dysfunction with good results and no significant side-effects [95, 96]. Moreover, non-invasive electrical stimulation systems such as transcutaneous electrical nerve stimulation (TENS) was highly effective in stimulating whole salivary flow in patients with xerostomia and hyposalivation caused by DM and postmenopausal condition [97, 98]. Acupuncture as a method of xerostomia treatment is also cited, a recent randomized and controlled pilot trial of acupuncture showed that acupuncture has beneficial effects on SS symptoms [99]. Other pilot study showed a preliminary evidence that auricular acupressure therapy may be effective in reducing xerostomia intensity in maintenance hemodialysis patients [100].

6.5. Glandular regeneration and gene therapy

Stem cell replacement therapy may be a good option to treat radiation-induced hyposalivation. Stem cell therapy attempts the repair of damaged salivary glands at the cellular level. In this regard, bone marrow stem cells, adipose tissue-derived stromal cells, dental pulp cells have been tested as a form of treatment for hyposalivation after radiotherapy [39]. Interestingly, human salivary stem/progenitor cells (hSSPCs) (derived from parotid and submandibular glands) can be cultured using the salisphere technique and can be introduced to a damaged salivary gland tissue to replace dead or damaged cells. In this context, Pringle et al. showed the presence of SSPCs in cultured human salipheres [101]. These cells were capable of self-renewal and differentiation, which when transplanted into irradiated recipients and restored glandular function. Considering that an ultimate goal is to develop fully functioning bioengineered organs to replace lost or damaged. It was recently reported that a population of SSPCs can be reliably isolated and expanded in sufficient number, suitable for use in a unique 3D hydrogel model of a human implantable salivary gland [102]. However, independent and collaborative work in stem cells research and tissue engineering is still necessary to have fully functional human salivary glands.

Gene therapy involves injecting a vector with genetic information into a tissue to result in some beneficial change. Originally, gene transfer was considered for use in treating congenital genetic disorders, but the basic principles have now been applied virtually to every organ, for acquired as well as inherited disorders. Regarding salivary glands, Baum et al., in phase I/II study, showed an increased saliva flow rate from the targeted parotid gland, as well as a reduction in symptoms related to the radiation-induced xerostomia in subjects treated with the transferring of cDNA for human aquaporin-1 (hAQP1) through an adenoviral (Ad5) vector (AdhAQP1) [103]. Additionally, others genes (Gli1, human keratinocyte growth factor, and Tousled like kinase 1B) have been targeted and have shown promise in preventing salivary hypofunction in a preclinical mouse [104, 105]. On the other hand, the use of small-interfering RNA (siRNA)-based gene silencing has provided protection of salivary gland from radiation-induced apoptosis at preclinical level [106].

7. Conclusion

Patients with xerostomia are often a challenge regarding diagnosis and treatment, because although xerostomia is not considered a disease, it has a potential devastating effect on the oral cavity. Since dentists are generally challenged with this problem, it is important to have an appropriate comprehension of diverse causes of xerostomia to develop a systematic approach that includes collaboration with physicians to facilitate interdisciplinary patient care, which involves its systemic conditions and medication. Furthermore, a comprehensive management of xerostomia is also necessary and it should incorporate patient education, lifestyle modifications, and adequate pharmacological and non-pharmacological therapies to improve the patient's quality of life. Since most of the successful therapies are depending on the parenchymal gland affection, it is essential to know new therapeutic approaches to fully recover *in vivo* the gland's function or to develop new bioengineered salivary tissues.

Acknowledgements

This work was supported by Faculty of Dentistry, University of Chile.

Author details

Alejandro Escobar[1]* and Juan P. Aitken-Saavedra[2,3]

*Address all correspondence to: janodvm@gmail.com

1 Institute for Research in Dental Sciences, Faculty of Dentistry, University of Chile, Santiago, Chile

2 Department of Oral Pathology and Medicine, Faculty of Dentistry, University of Chile, Santiago, Chile

3 Post Graduate Program in Dentistry, Federal University of Pelotas, Pelotas, Brazil

References

[1] Atkinson JC, Grisius M, Massey W. Salivary hypofunction and xerostomia: Diagnosis and treatment. Dental Clinics of North America. 2005;**49**:309-326. DOI: 10.1016/j.cden.2004.10.002

[2] Atkinson JC, Baum BJ. Salivary enhancement: Current status and future therapies. Journal of Dental Education. 2001;**65**:1096-1101

[3] Grisius MM. Salivary gland dysfunction: A review of systemic therapies. Oral Surgery, Oral Medicine, Oral Pathology, Oral Radiology, and Endodontics. 2001;**92**:156-162. DOI: 10.1067/moe.2001.116601

[4] Miranda-Rius J, Brunet-Llobet L, Lahor-Soler E, Farre M. Salivary secretory disorders, inducing drugs, and clinical management. International Journal of Medical Sciences. 2015; **12**:811-824. DOI: 10.7150/ijms.12912

[5] Porter SR, Scully C. Adverse drug reactions in the mouth. Clinics in Dermatology. 2000; **18**:525-532

[6] Wiener RC, Wu B, Crout R, Wiener M, Plassman B, Kao E, McNeil D. Hyposalivation and xerostomia in dentate older adults. Journal of the American Dental Association (1939). 2010;**141**:279-284

[7] Ship JA, Fox PC, Michalek JE, Cummins MJ, Richards AB. Treatment of primary Sjogren's syndrome with low-dose natural human interferon-alpha administered by the oral mucosal route: A phase II clinical trial. IFN Protocol Study Group. Journal of Interferon & Cytokine Research. 1999;**19**:943-951. DOI: 10.1089/107999099313497

[8] Gurvits GE, Tan A. Burning mouth syndrome. World Journal of Gastroenterology. 2013; **19**:665-672. DOI: 10.3748/wjg.v19.i5.665

[9] Bossola M, Tazza L. Xerostomia in patients on chronic hemodialysis. Nature Reviews. Nephrology. 2012;**8**:176-182. DOI: 10.1038/nrneph.2011.218

[10] Ivanovski K, Naumovski V, Kostadinova M, Pesevska S, Drijanska K, Filipce V. Xerostomia and salivary levels of glucose and urea in patients with diabetes. Prilozi. 2012;**33**: 219-229

[11] Tanasiewicz M, Hildebrandt T, Obersztyn I. Xerostomia of various etiologies: A review of the literature. Advances in Clinical and Experimental Medicine. 2016;**25**:199-206. DOI: 10.17219/acem/29375

[12] Napenas JJ, Brennan MT, Fox PC. Diagnosis and treatment of xerostomia (dry mouth). Odontology. 2009;**97**:76-83. DOI: 10.1007/s10266-008-0099-7

[13] Hopcraft MS, Tan C. Xerostomia: An update for clinicians. Australian Dental Journal. 2010;**55**:238-244. DOI: 10.1111/j.1834-7819.2010.01229.x. quiz 353

[14] Llena-Puy C. The role of saliva in maintaining oral health and as an aid to diagnosis. Medicina Oral, Patología Oral y Cirugía Bucal. 2006;**11**:E449-E455

[15] DJ O, Lee JY, Kim YK, Kho HS. Effects of carboxymethylcellulose (CMC)-based artificial saliva in patients with xerostomia. International Journal of Oral and Maxillofacial Surgery. 2008;**37**:1027-1031. DOI: 10.1016/j.ijom.2008.06.006

[16] Silvestre FJ, Minguez MP, Sune-Negre JM. Clinical evaluation of a new artificial saliva in spray form for patients with dry mouth. Medicina Oral, Patología Oral y Cirugía Bucal. 2009;**14**:E8-E11

[17] Shigeyama C, Ansai T, Awano S, Soh I, Yoshida A, Hamasaki T, Kakinoki Y, Tominaga K, Takahashi T, Takehara T. Salivary levels of cortisol and chromogranin A in patients with dry mouth compared with age-matched controls. Oral Surgery, Oral Medicine, Oral Pathology, Oral Radiology, and Endodontics. 2008;**106**:833-839

[18] Flink H, Bergdahl M, Tegelberg A, Rosenblad A, Lagerlof F. Prevalence of hyposalivation in relation to general health, body mass index and remaining teeth in different age groups of adults. Community Dentistry and Oral Epidemiology. 2008;**36**:523-531. DOI: 10.1111/j.1600-0528.2008.00432.x

[19] Dost F, Farah CS. Stimulating the discussion on saliva substitutes: A clinical perspective. Australian Dental Journal. 2013;**58**:11-17. DOI: 10.1111/adj.12023

[20] Femiano F, Rullo R, di Spirito F, Lanza A, Festa VM, Cirillo N. A comparison of salivary substitutes versus a natural sialogogue (citric acid) in patients complaining of dry mouth as an adverse drug reaction: A clinical, randomized controlled study. Oral Surgery, Oral Medicine, Oral Pathology, Oral Radiology, and Endodontics. 2011;**112**:e15-e20. DOI: 10.1016/j.tripleo.2011.01.039

[21] McMillan AS, Tsang CS, Wong MC, Kam AY. Efficacy of a novel lubricating system in the management of radiotherapy-related xerostomia. Oral Oncology. 2006;**42**:842-848. DOI: 10.1016/j.oraloncology.2005.12.003

[22] Tschoppe P, Wolf O, Eichhorn M, Martus P, Kielbassa AM. Design of a randomized controlled double-blind crossover clinical trial to assess the effects of saliva substitutes on bovine enamel and dentin in situ. BMC Oral Health. 2011;**11**:13. DOI: 10.1186/1472-6831-11-13

[23] Visvanathan V, Nix P. Managing the patient presenting with xerostomia: A review. International Journal of Clinical Practice. 2010;**64**:404-407. DOI: 10.1111/j.1742-1241.2009.02132.x

[24] Delli K, Spijkervet FK, Kroese FG, Bootsma H, Vissink A. Xerostomia. Monographs in Oral Science. 2014;**24**:109-125. DOI: 10.1159/000358792

[25] Chambers MS, Garden AS, Kies MS, Martin JW. Radiation-induced xerostomia in patients with head and neck cancer: Pathogenesis, impact on quality of life, and management. Head & Neck. 2004;**26**:796-807. DOI: 10.1002/hed.20045

[26] Singh M, Tonk RS. Xerostomia: Etiology, diagnosis, and management. Dentistry Today. 2012;**31**:80, 82-83; quiz 84-85

[27] Ugga L, Ravanelli M, Pallottino AA, Farina D, Maroldi R. Diagnostic work-up in obstructive and inflammatory salivary gland disorders. Acta Otorhinolaryngologica Italica. 2017;**37**:83-93. DOI: 10.14639/0392-100X-1597

[28] Fox PC, Busch KA, Baum BJ. Subjective reports of xerostomia and objective measures of salivary gland performance. Journal of the American Dental Association (1939). 1987;**115**:581-584

[29] Bascones-Martinez A, Munoz-Corcuera M, Bascones-Ilundain C. Side effects of drugs on the oral cavity. Medicina Clínica (Barcelona). 2015;**144**:126-131. DOI: 10.1016/j.medcli.2014.01.025

[30] Dodds MW, Johnson DA, Yeh CK. Health benefits of saliva: A review. Journal of Dentistry. 2005;**33**:223-233. DOI: 10.1016/j.jdent.2004.10.009

[31] Zero DT, Brennan MT, Daniels TE, Papas A, Stewart C, Pinto A, Al-Hashimi I, Navazesh M, Rhodus N, Sciubba J, Singh M, AJ W, Frantsve-Hawley J, Tracy S, Fox PC, Ford TL, Cohen S, Vivino FB, Hammitt KM. Clinical practice guidelines for oral management of Sjogren disease: Dental caries prevention. Journal of the American Dental Association (1939). 2016;**147**:295-305. DOI: 10.1016/j.adaj.2015.11.008

[32] Saavedra AJRM, Bozo MI, Ríos HM. Estudio de confiabilidad de la prueba de sialometría para flujo no estimulado en sujetos adultos clínicamente sanos. Revista Clínica de Periodoncia, Implantología y Rehabilitación Oral. 2013;**6**:25-28

[33] Berti-Couto Sde A, Couto-Souza PH, Jacobs R, Nackaerts O, Rubira-Bullen IR, Westphalen FH, Moyses SJ, Ignacio SA, Costa MB, Tolazzi AL. Clinical diagnosis of hyposalivation in hospitalized patients. Journal of Applied Oral Science. 2012;**20**:157-161

[34] Ergun S, Cekici A, Topcuoglu N, Migliari DA, Kulekci G, Tanyeri H, Isik G. Oral status and *Candida* colonization in patients with Sjogren's Syndrome. Medicina Oral, Patología Oral y Cirugía Bucal. 2010;**15**:e310-e315

[35] Mungia R, Cano SM, Johnson DA, Dang H, Brown JP. Interaction of age and specific saliva component output on caries. Aging Clinical and Experimental Research. 2008;**20**:503-508

[36] Jensen SB, Pedersen AM, Vissink A, Andersen E, Brown CG, Davies AN, Dutilh J, Fulton JS, Jankovic L, Lopes NN, Mello AL, Muniz LV, Murdoch-Kinch CA, Nair RG, Napenas JJ, Nogueira-Rodrigues A, Saunders D, Stirling B, von Bultzingslowen I, Weikel DS, Elting LS, Spijkervet FK, Brennan MT. A systematic review of salivary gland hypofunction and xerostomia induced by cancer therapies: Prevalence, severity and impact on quality of life. Supportive Care in Cancer. 2010;**18**:1039-1060. DOI: 10.1007/s00520-010-0827-8

[37] Navazesh M, Christensen C, Brightman V. Clinical criteria for the diagnosis of salivary gland hypofunction. Journal of Dental Research. 1992;**71**:1363-1369. DOI: 10.1177/00220345920710070301

[38] Aitken-Saavedra J, Rojas-Alcayaga G, Maturana-Ramirez A, Escobar-Alvarez A, Cortes-Coloma A, Reyes-Rojas M, Viera-Sapiain V, Villablanca-Martinez C, Morales-Bozo I. Salivary gland dysfunction markers in type 2 diabetes mellitus patients. Journal of Clinical and Experimental Dentistry. 2015;**7**:e501-e505. DOI: 10.4317/jced.52329

[39] Saleh J, Figueiredo MA, Cherubini K, Salum FG. Salivary hypofunction: An update on a etiology, diagnosis and therapeutics. Archives of Oral Biology. 2015;**60**:242-255. DOI: 10.1016/j.archoralbio.2014.10.004

[40] Tylenda CA, Ship JA, Fox PC, Baum BJ. Evaluation of submandibular salivary flow rate in different age groups. Journal of Dental Research. 1988;**67**:1225-1228. DOI: 10.1177/00220345880670091501

[41] Yeh CK, Johnson DA, Dodds MW. Impact of aging on human salivary gland function: A community-based study. Aging (Milano). 1998;**10**:421-428

[42] Smith CH, Boland B, Daureeawoo Y, Donaldson E, Small K, Tuomainen J. Effect of aging on stimulated salivary flow in adults. Journal of the American Geriatrics Society. 2013;**61**:805-808. DOI: 10.1111/jgs.12219

[43] Mese H, Matsuo R. Salivary secretion, taste and hyposalivation. Journal of Oral Rehabilitation. 2007;**34**:711-723. DOI: 10.1111/j.1365-2842.2007.01794.x

[44] Ettinger RL. Review: Xerostomia: A symptom which acts like a disease. Age and Ageing. 1996;**25**:409, 412

[45] Kumar NN, Panchaksharappa MG, Annigeri RG. Modified schirmer test—A screening tool for xerostomia among subjects on antidepressants. Archives of Oral Biology. 2014;**59**:829-834. DOI: 10.1016/j.archoralbio.2014.05.008

[46] Uher R, Farmer A, Henigsberg N, Rietschel M, Mors O, Maier W, Kozel D, Hauser J, Souery D, Placentino A, Strohmaier J, Perroud N, Zobel A, Rajewska-Rager A, Dernovsek MZ, Larsen ER, Kalember P, Giovannini C, Barreto M, McGuffin P, Aitchison KJ. Adverse reactions to antidepressants. The British Journal of Psychiatry. 2009;**195**:202-210. DOI: 10.1192/bjp.bp.108.061960

[47] Diaz-Arnold AM, Marek CA. The impact of saliva on patient care: A literature review. The Journal of Prosthetic Dentistry. 2002;**88**:337, 343

[48] Navazesh M, Brightman VJ, Pogoda JM. Relationship of medical status, medications, and salivary flow rates in adults of different ages. Oral Surgery, Oral Medicine, Oral Pathology, Oral Radiology, and Endodontics. 1996;**81**:172-176

[49] Sreebny LM, Yu A, Green A, Valdini A. Xerostomia in diabetes mellitus. Diabetes Care. 1992;**15**:900-904

[50] Dirix P, Nuyts S, Van den Bogaert W. Radiation-induced xerostomia in patients with head and neck cancer: A literature review. Cancer. 2006;**107**:2525-2534. DOI: 10.1002/cncr.22302

[51] Shannon IL, Trodahl JN, Starcke EN. Radiosensitivity of the human parotid gland. Proceedings of the Society for Experimental Biology and Medicine. 1978;**157**:50-53

[52] Lasisi TJ, Fasanmade AA. Salivary flow and composition in diabetic and non-diabetic subjects. Nigerian Journal of Physiological Sciences. 2012;**27**:79-82

[53] Bagheri H, Damase-Michel C, Lapeyre-Mestre M, Cismondo S, O'Connell D, Senard JM, Rascol O, Montastruc JL. A study of salivary secretion in Parkinson's disease. Clinical Neuropharmacology. 1999;**22**:213-215

[54] Proulx M, de Courval FP, Wiseman MA, Panisset M. Salivary production in Parkinson's disease. Movement Disorders. 2005;**20**:204-207. DOI: 10.1002/mds.20189

[55] Bergdahl M, Bergdahl J, Johansson I. Depressive symptoms in individuals with idiopathic subjective dry mouth. Journal of Oral Pathology & Medicine. 1997;**26**:448-450

[56] Anttila SS, Knuuttila ML, Sakki TK. Depressive symptoms as an underlying factor of the sensation of dry mouth. Psychosomatic Medicine. 1998;**60**:215-218

[57] Ahmad MS, Bhayat A, Zafar MS, Al-Samadani KH. The impact of hyposalivation on quality of life (QoL) and oral health in the aging population of Al Madinah Al Munawarrah. International Journal of Environmental Research and Public Health. 2017;**14**, **445**:1-11. DOI: 10.3390/ijerph14040445

[58] Deng J, Jackson L, Epstein JB, Migliorati CA, Murphy BA. Dental demineralization and caries in patients with head and neck cancer. Oral Oncology. 2015;**51**:824-831. DOI: 10.1016/j.oraloncology.2015.06.009

[59] Paranhos Hde F, Salles AE, Macedo LD, Silva-Lovato CH, Pagnano VO, Watanabe E. Complete denture biofilm after brushing with specific denture paste, neutral soap and artificial saliva. Brazilian Dental Journal. 2013;**24**:47-52

[60] Billings M, Dye BA, Iafolla T, Grisius M, Alevizos I. Elucidating the role of hyposalivation and autoimmunity in oral candidiasis. Oral Diseases. 2017;**23**:387-394. DOI: 10.1111/odi.12626

[61] Plemons JM, Al-Hashimi I, Marek CL. Managing xerostomia and salivary gland hypofunction: Executive summary of a report from the American Dental Association Council on Scientific Affairs. Journal of the American Dental Association (1939). 2014;**145**:867-873. DOI: 10.14219/jada.2014.44

[62] Andreassen CN, Grau C, Lindegaard JC. Chemical radioprotection: A critical review of amifostine as a cytoprotector in radiotherapy. Seminars in Radiation Oncology. 2003;**13**:62-72. DOI: 10.1053/srao.2003.50006

[63] Yuhas JM. A more general role for WR-2721 in cancer therapy. British Journal of Cancer. 1980;**41**:832-834

[64] Nagler RM, Baum BJ. Prophylactic treatment reduces the severity of xerostomia following radiation therapy for oral cavity cancer. Archives of Otolaryngology – Head & Neck Surgery. 2003;**129**:247-250

[65] Riley P, Glenny AM, Hua F, Worthington HV. Pharmacological interventions for preventing dry mouth and salivary gland dysfunction following radiotherapy. Cochrane Database of Systematic Reviews. 2017;**7**:CD012744. DOI: 10.1002/14651858.CD012744

[66] Wasserman TH, Brizel DM, Henke M, Monnier A, Eschwege F, Sauer R, Strnad V. Influence of intravenous amifostine on xerostomia, tumor control, and survival after radiotherapy for head-and-neck cancer: 2-year follow-up of a prospective, randomized, phase III trial. International Journal of Radiation Oncology, Biology, Physics. 2005;**63**:985-990. DOI: 10.1016/j.ijrobp.2005.07.966

[67] Choi JS, Shin HS, An HY, Kim YM, Lim JY. Radioprotective effects of Keratinocyte Growth Factor-1 against irradiation-induced salivary gland hypofunction. Oncotarget. 2017;**8**:13496-13508. DOI: 10.18632/oncotarget.14583

[68] Brizel DM, Murphy BA, Rosenthal DI, Pandya KJ, Gluck S, Brizel HE, Meredith RF, Berger D, Chen MG, Mendenhall W. Phase II study of palifermin and concurrent chemoradiation in head and neck squamous cell carcinoma. Journal of Clinical Oncology. 2008;**26**:2489-2496. DOI: 10.1200/JCO.2007.13.7349

[69] Liu R, Seikaly H, Jha N. Anatomic study of submandibular gland transfer in an attempt to prevent postradiation xerostomia. The Journal of Otolaryngology. 2002;**31**:76-79

[70] Jha N, Seikaly H, Harris J, Williams D, Liu R, McGaw T, Hofmann H, Robinson D, Hanson J, Barnaby P. Prevention of Radiation Induced Xerostomia by Surgical Transfer of Submandibular Salivary Gland Into the Submental Space. 2003. Available from: http://www.ncbi.nlm.nih.gov/pubmed/12742268

[71] Dalodom S, Lam-Ubol A, Jeanmaneechotechai S, Takamfoo L, Intachai W, Duangchada K, Hongsachum B, Kanjanatiwat P, Vacharotayangul P, Trachootham D. Influence of oral moisturizing jelly as a saliva substitute for the relief of xerostomia in elderly patients with hypertension and diabetes mellitus. Geriatric Nursing. 2016;**37**:101-109. DOI: 10.1016/j.gerinurse.2015.10.014

[72] Hahnel S, Behr M, Handel G, Burgers R. Saliva substitutes for the treatment of radiation-induced xerostomia—A review. Supportive Care in Cancer. 2009;**17**:1331-1343. DOI: 10.1007/s00520-009-0671-x

[73] Vissink A, s-Gravenmade EJ, Panders AK, Vermey A, Petersen JK, Visch LL, Schaub RM. A clinical comparison between commercially available mucin- and CMC-containing saliva substitutes. International Journal of Oral Surgery. 1983;**12**:232-238

[74] Epstein JB, Villines DC, Singh M, Papas A. Management of dry mouth: Assessment of oral symptoms after use of a polysaccharide-based oral rinse. Oral Surgery, Oral Medicine, Oral Pathology, Oral Radiology. 2017;**123**:76-83. DOI: 10.1016/j.oooo.2016.09.008

[75] Navarro Morante A, Wolff A, Bautista Mendoza GR, Lopez-Jornet P. Natural products for the management of xerostomia: A randomized, double-blinded, placebo-controlled clinical trial. Journal of Oral Pathology & Medicine. 2017;**46**:154-160. DOI: 10.1111/jop.12487

[76] Regelink G, Vissink A, Reintsema H, Nauta JM. Efficacy of a synthetic polymer saliva substitute in reducing oral complaints of patients suffering from irradiation-induced xerostomia. Quintessence International. 1998;**29**:383-388

[77] Barbe AG, Schmidt-Park Y, Hamacher S, Derman SH, Noack MJ. Efficacy of GUM(R) Hydral versus Biotene(R) Oralbalance mouthwashes plus gels on symptoms of medication-induced xerostomia: A randomized, double-blind, crossover study. Clinical Oral Investigations. 2018;**22**:169-180. DOI: 10.1007/s00784-017-2096-0

[78] Saavedra JM, Juorio AV, Shigematsu K, Pinto JE. Specific insulin binding sites in snail (*Helix aspersa*) ganglia. Cellular and Molecular Neurobiology. 1989;**9**:273-279

[79] Tsibouklis J, Middleton AM, Patel N, Pratten J. Toward mucoadhesive hydrogel formulations for the management of xerostomia: The physicochemical, biological, and pharmacological considerations. Journal of Biomedical Materials Research. Part A. 2013;**101**:3327-3338. DOI: 10.1002/jbm.a.34626

[80] Gurkar H, Venkatesh OY, Somashekar JM, Gowda MH, Dwivedi M, Ningthoujam I. Prosthodontic management of xerostomic patient: A technical modification. Case Reports in Dentistry. 2016;**2016**:8905891. DOI: 10.1155/2016/8905891

[81] Gotrick B, Akerman S, Ericson D, Torstenson R, Tobin G. Oral pilocarpine for treatment of opioid-induced oral dryness in healthy adults. Journal of Dental Research. 2004;**83**:393-397. DOI: 10.1177/154405910408300508

[82] Fox PC, Atkinson JC, Macynski AA, Wolff A, Kung DS, Valdez IH, Jackson W, Delapenha RA, Shiroky J, Baum BJ. Pilocarpine treatment of salivary gland hypofunction and dry mouth (xerostomia). Archives of Internal Medicine. 1991;**151**:1149-1152

[83] Weber J, Keating GM. Cevimeline. Drugs. 2008;**68**:1691-1698

[84] Chambers MS, Posner M, Jones CU, Biel MA, Hodge KM, Vitti R, Armstrong I, Yen C, Weber RS. Cevimeline for the treatment of postirradiation xerostomia in patients with head and neck cancer. International Journal of Radiation Oncology, Biology, Physics. 2007;**68**:1102-1109. DOI: 10.1016/j.ijrobp.2007.01.019

[85] Everett HC. The use of bethanechol chloride with tricyclic antidepressants. The American Journal of Psychiatry. 1975;**132**:1202-1204. DOI: 10.1176/ajp.132.11.1202

[86] Fossaluzza V. Bromhexine in symptomatic treatment of Sjogren syndrome. Klinische Monatsblätter für Augenheilkunde. 1984;**185**:292-295. DOI: 10.1055/s-2008-1054619

[87] Ichikawa Y, Tokunaga M, Shimizu H, Moriuchi J, Takaya M, Arimori S. Clinical trial of ambroxol (Mucosolvan) in Sjogren's syndrome. The Tokai Journal of Experimental and Clinical Medicine. 1988;**13**:165-169

[88] Adachi K, Ono M, Kawamura A, Yuki M, Fujishiro H, Kinoshita Y. Nizatidine and cisapride enhance salivary secretion in humans. Alimentary Pharmacology & Therapeutics. 2002;**16**:297-301

[89] Nin T, Umemoto M, Negoro A, Miuchi S, Sakagami M. Nizatidine enhances salivary secretion in patients with dry mouth. Auris, Nasus, Larynx. 2008;**35**:224-229. DOI: 10.1016/j.anl.2007.08.002

[90] Khurshudian AV. A pilot study to test the efficacy of oral administration of interferon-alpha lozenges to patients with Sjogren's syndrome. Oral Surgery, Oral Medicine, Oral Pathology, Oral Radiology, and Endodontics. 2003;**95**:38-44. DOI: 10.1067/moe.2003.30

[91] Steinfeld SD, Demols P, Appelboom T. Infliximab in primary Sjogren's syndrome: One-year followup. Arthritis and Rheumatism. 2002;**46**:3301-3303. DOI: 10.1002/art.10674

[92] Fox PC. Salivary enhancement therapies. Caries Research. 2004;**38**:241-246. DOI: 10.1159/000077761

[93] Itthagarun A, Wei SH. Chewing gum and saliva in oral health. The Journal of Clinical Dentistry. 1997;**8**:159-162

[94] Van Loveren C. Sugar alcohols: What is the evidence for caries-preventive and caries-therapeutic effects? Caries Research. 2004;**38**:286-293. DOI: 10.1159/000077768

[95] Alajbeg I, Falcao DP, Tran SD, Martin-Granizo R, Lafaurie GI, Matranga D, Pejda S, Vuletic L, Mantilla R, Leal SC, Bezerra AC, Menard HA, Kimoto S, Pan S, Maniegas L, Krushinski CA, Melilli D, Campisi G, Paderni C, Mendoza GR, Yepes JF, Lindh L, Koray M, Mumcu G, Elad S, Zeevi I, Barrios BC, Lopez Sanchez RM, Lassauzay C, Fromentin O, Beiski BZ, Strietzel FP, Konttinen YT, Wolff A, Zunt SL. Intraoral electrostimulator for xerostomia relief: A long-term, multicenter, open-label, uncontrolled, clinical trial. Oral Surgery, Oral Medicine, Oral Pathology, Oral Radiology. 2012;**113**:773-781. DOI: 10.1016/j.oooo.2012.01.012

[96] Strietzel FP, Lafaurie GI, Mendoza GR, Alajbeg I, Pejda S, Vuletic L, Mantilla R, Falcao DP, Leal SC, Bezerra AC, Tran SD, Menard HA, Kimoto S, Pan S, Martin-Granizo RA, Lozano ML, Zunt SL, Krushinski CA, Melilli D, Campisi G, Paderni C, Dolce S, Yepes JF, Lindh L, Koray M, Mumcu G, Elad S, Zeevi I, Barrios BC, Lopez Sanchez RM, Beiski BZ, Wolff A, Konttinen YT. Efficacy and safety of an intraoral electrostimulation device for xerostomia relief: A multicenter, randomized trial. Arthritis and Rheumatism. 2011;**63**:180-190. DOI: 10.1002/art.27766

[97] Dyasnoor S, Kamath S, Khader NFA. Effectiveness of electrostimulation on whole salivary flow among patients with type 2 diabetes mellitus. The Permanente Journal. 2017;**21**:15-164. DOI: 10.7812/TPP/15-164

[98] Konidena A, Sharma D, Puri G, Dixit A, Jatti D, Gupta R. Effect of TENS on stimulation of saliva in postmenopausal women with or without oral dryness—An interventional study. Journal of Oral Biology and Craniofacial Research. 2016;**6**:S44-S50. DOI: 10.1016/j.jobcr.2016.01.004

[99] Jiang Q, Zhang H, Pang R, Chen J, Liu Z, Zhou X. Acupuncture for primary Sjogren syndrome (pSS) on symptomatic improvements: Study protocol for a randomized controlled trial. BMC Complementary and Alternative Medicine. 2017;**17**:61. DOI: 10.1186/s12906-017-1559-9

[100] Yang G, Lin S, Wu Y, Zhang S, Wu X, Liu X, Zou C, Lin Q. Auricular acupressure helps alleviate xerostomia in maintenance hemodialysis patients: A pilot study. Journal of Alternative and Complementary Medicine. 2017;**23**:278-284. DOI: 10.1089/acm.2016.0283

[101] Pringle S, Maimets M, van der Zwaag M, Stokman MA, van Gosliga D, Zwart E, Witjes MJ, de Haan G, van Os R, Coppes RP. Human salivary gland stem cells functionally restore radiation damaged salivary glands. Stem Cells. 2016;**34**:640-652. DOI: 10.1002/stem.2278

[102] Srinivasan PP, Patel VN, Liu S, Harrington DA, Hoffman MP, Jia X, Witt RL, Farach-Carson MC, Pradhan-Bhatt S. Primary salivary human stem/progenitor cells undergo microenvironment-driven Acinar-like differentiation in hyaluronate hydrogel culture. Stem Cells Translational Medicine. 2017;**6**:110-120. DOI: 10.5966/sctm.2016-0083

[103] Baum BJ, Alevizos I, Zheng C, Cotrim AP, Liu S, McCullagh L, Goldsmith CM, Burbelo PD, Citrin DE, Mitchell JB, Nottingham LK, Rudy SF, Van Waes C, Whatley MA, Brahim JS, Chiorini JA, Danielides S, Turner RJ, Patronas NJ, Chen CC, Nikolov NP, Illei GG. Early responses to adenoviral-mediated transfer of the aquaporin-1 cDNA for radiation-induced salivary hypofunction. Proceedings of the National Academy of Sciences of the United States of America. 2012;**109**:19403-19407. DOI: 10.1073/pnas.1210662109

[104] Hai B, Qin L, Yang Z, Zhao Q, Shangguan L, Ti X, Zhao Y, Kim S, Rangaraj D, Liu F. Transient activation of hedgehog pathway rescued irradiation-induced hyposalivation by preserving salivary stem/progenitor cells and parasympathetic innervation. Clinical Cancer Research. 2014;**20**:140-150. DOI: 10.1158/1078-0432.CCR-13-1434

[105] Palaniyandi S, Odaka Y, Green W, Abreo F, Caldito G, De Benedetti A, Sunavala-Dossabhoy G. Adenoviral delivery of tousled kinase for the protection of salivary glands against ionizing radiation damage. Gene Therapy. 2011;**18**:275-282. DOI: 10.1038/gt.2010.142

[106] Arany S, Benoit DS, Dewhurst S, Ovitt CE. Nanoparticle-mediated gene silencing confers radioprotection to salivary glands in vivo. Molecular Therapy. 2013;**21**:1182-1194. DOI: 10.1038/mt.2013.42

Chapter 3

Sialorrhea: A Guide to Etiology, Assessment, and Management

Işıl Adadan Güvenç

Additional information is available at the end of the chapter

http://dx.doi.org/10.5772/intechopen.82619

Abstract

Sialorrhea, also known as hypersalivation or ptyalism, is excessive salivation associated with neurological disorders or localized anatomical abnormalities in the oral cavity. Pathologic sialorrhea may develop due to hypersalivation, together with various neurologic disorders including cerebral palsy, Parkinson's disease, and amyotrophic lateral sclerosis, or as an adverse effect of medications. Sialorrhea results in numerous problematic physical and psychosocial complications and has a significant negative impact on quality of life for both the patient and caregiver. The management of sialorrhea is best accomplished with a multidisciplinary team approach. Treatment options range from conservative measures such as observation, positioning, behavioral therapies, and pharmacological therapy to more aggressive methods such as botulinum toxin injections or surgery. The physiology, etiology, assessment, and treatment of sialorrhea are outlined in this review.

Keywords: sialorrhea, hypersalivation, drooling, ptyalism, etiology, assessment, management

1. Introduction

Sialorrhea, also known as hypersalivation or ptyalism, is excessive salivation associated with neurological disorders or localized anatomical abnormalities in the oral cavity. Sialorrhea can be classified as anterior and posterior; both can occur separately or simultaneously. Posterior sialorrhea is the flowing of saliva from the tongue to the pharynx. Anterior sialorrhea results in salivary incontinence or involuntary spillage of saliva over the lower lip, known as drooling. The underlying etiology is the excessive production of saliva or inability to retain saliva within the mouth due to reduced neuromuscular control of the tongue, oral tissues, and impairment in the swallowing mechanism, all of which are necessary to move saliva from the oral cavity to the oropharynx and beyond [1]. Drooling is common in normally developed babies but subsides between the ages 15 and 36 months with the establishment of salivary continence. Sialorrhea after 4 years of age is generally considered pathologic. Pathologic sialorrhea may develop due to hypersalivation, together with numerous neurologic disorders including cerebral palsy (CP), Parkinson's disease (PD), and amyotrophic lateral sclerosis (ALS), or as an adverse effect of medications. In children, the most common cause of sialorrhea is CP, which persists in 10–38% of these patients. In adults, the most common cause of sialorrhea is PD with a rate of 70–80% [2].

Whatever the cause is, drooling is bothersome, resulting in physical and psychosocial complications. Physical complications include maceration of the skin around the mouth with secondary infection, bad odor, dehydration, speech disturbance, and interference with feeding. People with drooling are also at increased risk for aspiration of saliva, food, or fluids into lungs, particularly when the normal reflex mechanisms such as gagging or coughing are impaired. The psychosocial complications include isolation, barriers to education (such as an inability to share books or computer keyboards), increased dependency and level of care, damage to electronic devices, decreased self-esteem, and difficult social interaction [3]. Sialorrhea may have a significant negative impact on quality of life for both the patient and caregiver [1].

2. Physiology of salivation

The major salivary glands include parotid, submandibular, and sublingual glands; the largest being the parotid gland. These glands secrete saliva, which has a major role in lubrication, digestion, immunity, and maintenance of homeostasis in the human body [2]. The salivary secretion of parotid, submandibular, and sublingual glands is controlled mainly by parasympathetic nervous system, although sympathetic innervation has a minor influence. The parasympathetic fibers originate in the pons and medulla, and they synapse in the otic and submandibular ganglia. Postganglionic fibers originating from the otic ganglion regulate secretory functions of the parotid gland, while the postganglionic fibers from the submandibular ganglion regulate secretory function of the submandibular and sublingual glands. Sympathetic innervation of these glands results in contraction of muscle fibers around the salivary ducts, which enhances the flow of saliva [3].

Salivary secretion is regulated through a reflex arch that produces several actions. The afferent branch contains chemoreceptors in taste buds and mechanoreceptors in the periodontal ligament. Afferent innervations of cranial nerves V, VII, IX, and X carry impulses to salivary nuclei in the medulla oblongata. Efferent impulses are mainly parasympathetic as described above; they come from the chorda tympani nerve (a branch of the cranial nerve VII) and travel to the submandibular, sublingual, and other minor glands via lingual nerve (a branch of the cranial nerve V_3). Efferent fibers to the parotid gland are supplied by lesser petrosal nerve (a branch of cranial nerve IX), which travel through the fibers of auriculotemporal nerve (a branch of the cranial nerve V_3) and reach the gland [2].

http://dx.doi.org/10.5772/intechopen.82619

The major salivary glands provide 90% of the nearly 1.5 L of saliva that is produced every day. If salivary secretion is not stimulated, that is in basal state, 70% of total salivary secretion comes from the submandibular and sublingual glands. When stimulated, salivary secretion increases by five times, with the parotid glands delivering the greater amount of the saliva [3]. An example of an exogenous source causing stimulation is chewing [2]. There are two main types of saliva produced by the three major salivary glands; serous saliva is produced mainly by parotid glands by stimulation, which is thin and watery, while viscous saliva is produced by sublingual and submandibular glands throughout the day, which is thicker [4]. Both forms of these secretions can be problematic. Serous saliva results in watery saliva, consistently spilling from the side of the mouth, and viscous saliva may be mucoid and sticky, which makes it harder to clear and causes a sensation of choking, associated with panic. It is important to distinguish between thin, runny saliva and thick, mucous secretions because the treatment options differ. The stimulation of cholinergic receptors produces thin, serous secretions, whereas that of beta-adrenergic receptors produces thick protein and mucus-rich secretions. Therefore, in the case of watery saliva secretions, anticholinergics can be preferred, whereas for thick mucus secretions, the addition of beta blockers may be beneficial [5].

3. Etiology of sialorrhea

Sialorrhea associated with neurologic illnesses is generally caused by impaired swallowing due to impaired neuromuscular function. Efficient coordination of various structures, namely the oral cavity, pharynx, larynx, and esophagus, is required for the neuromuscular activity of swallowing. The coordination of these structures forms three phases; the oral phase is under voluntary control, followed by the pharyngeal and esophageal phases, which are involuntary. Spontaneous swallowing is essential for the control of drooling. In children with neurologic disorders, drooling is similarly the result of inefficient tongue and/or bulbar control, thus impaired swallowing, rather than hypersalivation [2].

In children, mental retardation and CP are the most common causes of sialorrhea. Roughly, one in three children with CP is reported to have some degree of sialorrhea. Sialorrhea in CP is caused by oral motor dysfunction, dysphagia, and intraoral sensitivity disorder. Though underestimated, sialorrhea has significant clinical and social consequences concerning the overall health of these children, including dysphagia, respiratory health, and socioemotional aspects of both the children and their caregivers [4]. In adults, PD is the most common etiology. Swallowing impairment, mostly in the oropharyngeal phase, is the major contributor to the pathophysiology of sialorrhea in PD patients, while an increase in the speed of salivary excretion might be a minor contributor. No increase in salivary production was demonstrated in scintigraphic studies in PD patients with sialorrhea, while the speed of salivary excretion of parotid glands in PD patients was significantly higher than normal controls with Tc-99 m scintigraphy [6]. Similarly, in ALS, sialorrhea is not caused by increased production of saliva, but by the inability to swallow secretions because of tongue spasticity, weakness of face, mouth and pharyngeal muscles, and loss of oropharyngeal coordination and function [5]. Less common neurologic causes of sialorrhea are pseudobulbar palsy, bulbar palsy, and stroke (**Table 1**).

Systemic causes

- Neuromuscular/sensory dysfunction—cerebral palsy, Parkinson's disease, mental retardation, motor neuron disease (ALS), pseudobulbar/bulbar palsy, stroke
- Medication side effects—antipsychotics (clozapine), tranquilizers, anticonvulsants, anticholinesterases, lithium
- Toxin exposure—mercury vapor, pesticides, snake poisoning, mushrooms
- Infection—rabies
- Gastric—gastroesophageal reflux

Local causes

- Oral Inflammation—teething
- Infection—dental caries, oral cavity infection, tonsillitis, peritonsillar abscess
- Anatomic—macroglossia, nasal blockage, oral incompetence, dental malocclusion, orthodontic problems, head and neck surgical defects

Physiological causes

- Pregnancy

Table 1. Etiology of sialorrhea.

Increased secretion of saliva frequently develops due to inflammation, such as teething, dental caries, and oral cavity infections. Pregnancy is another significant cause of hypersecretion, usually related to hyperemesis gravidarum. It has an abrupt onset in the 2nd and 3rd week of conception with the rise of hormones and usually resolves during 2nd trimester [7]. Other causes of hypersecretion include side effects from medications (i.e., antipsychotics, tranquilizers, anticonvulsants, cholinergic agonists, and lithium), gastroesophageal reflux, toxin exposure (i.e., mercury vapor, poisonous spider bites, mushrooms, insecticides), and rabies [3, 8]. Clozapine, an antipsychotic used in schizophrenia, is a rather common cause of sialorrhea, which manifests in 30–80% of patients taking the drug. Hypersalivation usually develops early in the treatment course and is typically more prominent at night [9].

Anatomic abnormalities are usually not the only cause of sialorrhea; however, most of the time, they exacerbate other causative conditions. Macroglossia (enlarged tongue) and oral incompetence may cause salivary spilling. A constantly open mouth due to nasal blockage or malocclusion and other orthodontic problems may compound oral incompetence; treatment of nasal problems and orthodontic correction can alleviate sialorrhea. Surgical defects occurring after major head and neck surgeries may result in sialorrhea as well [3].

4. Assessment of sialorrhea

Assessment of the severity of sialorrhea and its impact on the quality of life for the patient and the caregivers assist in establishing a prognosis and appropriate management of the problem. History should be taken from the patient and the caregiver to understand the etiology and severity of the situation and its impact on the daily life. Use of medications, language and communication skills, cognition, respiratory health, and presence of gastroesophageal reflux disease should be questioned. In physical examination, oral cavity should be examined for sores on the lip and chin, dental problems, tongue size and movement, and tonsillar

Drooling severity	Points
Dry (never drools)	1
Mild (wet lips only)	2
Moderate (wet lips and chin)	3
Severe (clothing becomes damp)	4
Profuse (clothing, hands, tray, objects become wet)	5
Drooling frequency	
Never drools	1
Occasionally drools	2
Frequently drools	3
Constantly drools	4

Table 2. Drooling frequency and severity scale.

hypertrophy; nasal blockage, malocclusion, and jaw stability should be assessed. A neurological examination should be carried out investigating the level of alertness, swallowing ability, motor skills, and sensory dysfunction of the patient. The nutrition and hydration status, head posture, and emotional state of the patient should also be evaluated [4, 10].

Objective and subjective measures have been developed to quantify sialorrhea. The objective test methods include radioisotope scanning, collection cups strapped to the patient's chin for the measurement of salivary flow, and direct observation of saliva loss such as counting the number of napkins used daily to contain excessive saliva production, measuring the weight of the towels or dental cotton rolls [4, 10]. The importance of objective methods is that they seem to be more sensitive in detecting a reduction in sialorrhea or drooling than purely subjective assessments [11].

A variety of subjective scales for sialorrhea have been described. Subjective scales such as the drooling frequency and severity scale, the drooling rating scale, the drooling impact Scale, and visual analog scales can be given to patients or their caregivers to determine the qualitative and quantitative consequences of the severity and impact of sialorrhea [4]. The drooling frequency and severity scale is an easy comprehensive scale, which rates the severity of drooling on a five-point scale and the frequency of drooling on a four-point scale (**Table 2**) [12]. Subjective scales are useful and appropriate methods to measure changes in sialorrhea, because the impact on families, caregivers, and the patients themselves is of utmost importance when assessing satisfaction with the effectiveness of any treatment [4].

5. Management of sialorrhea

The management of sialorrhea continues to be a challenge in spite of various effective treatment strategies to diminish saliva production. The flow of saliva from the oral cavity to the esophagus depends on numerous factors, such as cognitive and mental abilities, intact swallowing, oral sensibility, lip closure, and ability to keep the head upright [1].

Treatment of sialorrhea is best accomplished with a multidisciplinary team approach. The complete history and physical examination of the patient, the assessment of the impact of drooling on quality of life, and the potential for improvement can be undertaken by the primary care physicians. Speech pathologists and occupational therapists provide education for swallowing mechanics to the patients and support their posture with devices such as the head back wheelchair. Dentists and orthodontists identify and correct dental and oral diseases and malocclusion. Otolaryngologists diagnose and treat causes of aerodigestive obstruction like macroglossia and adenotonsillar hypertrophy that contribute to drooling. Neurologists assess the severity and prognosis of neurologic conditions that result in drooling [3].

The goal of the treatment of drooling is a reduction in excessive salivary flow, while maintaining a moist and healthy oral cavity. Avoidance of xerostomia (dry mouth) is essential. The two main approaches are:

1. Noninvasive modalities including positioning, improving eating and drinking skills, oral facial facilitation, speech therapy, biofeedback, positive and negative reinforcement, oral prosthetic devices, pharmacological therapy, and botulinum toxin
2. Invasive modalities including surgery and radiotherapy

Generally, no single approach is adequately effective, and usually, a combination of therapies is used. Primarily, reversible causes of drooling should be treated. Less invasive and reversible methods are preferred before surgery is undertaken [10]. Behavioral approaches and therapies employed by speech pathologists are rarely curative, while systemic medications and surgical approaches may have severe and long-term adverse effects [1].

For minimal problems, in children younger than 4 years of age or in adults with unstable neurologic function, observation may be the convenient choice. Minimal issues can be handled with a feeding program aimed at improving oral-motor control as well; nevertheless, this can rarely be helpful. Anatomical problems should be identified and treated, and adenotonsillectomy should be undertaken, if necessary. Dental malocclusion and caries should be corrected. Patients should be fitted with appropriate wheelchairs and braces, when required. A number of orthodontic appliances may be used, such as customized plates that fit the palate for improving lip closure or movable beads placed on the upper plate that stimulate tongue movement, thus helping to deflect saliva toward the pharynx [3].

Other conservative therapeutic options include positioning techniques, oral-motor, and speech therapies given by speech therapists, which improve oral awareness and motor control. Biofeedback and automatic cueing techniques may be utilized in patients with mild neurologic dysfunction and drooling. These devices are used to associate a behavior with a cue, such as swallowing or wiping the face with a beep sound. Reinforcement methods, which are suggested behaviors such as encouraging patients for swallowing and wiping their faces and discouraging open mouth, can be used as an adjunct in moderate sialorrhea [3, 10].

Whenever sialorrhea continues to affect the patient's health and quality of life in spite of these conservative measures, pharmacological therapy and other invasive therapies should be considered.

5.1. Pharmacological therapy

Oral therapy for sialorrhea encompasses the use of anticholinergic agents such as glycopyrrolate, benztropine, scopolamine, and tropicamide. Anticholinergic agents work by downregulating acetylcholine and ultimately decreasing saliva secretion through the parasympathetic autonomic nervous system. Glycopyrrolate oral solution is an anticholinergic agent that was the first drug approved in the United States for drooling in children with neurologic conditions and is generally well tolerated. However, anticholinergic agents are poorly tolerated by elderly patients. Glycopyrrolate actually has lower risk of central side effects, owing to its quaternary ammonium structure, that makes it impossible to pass the blood–brain barrier in large amounts. It is effective and safe at 1 mg, 3 times a day [2]. Studies have shown 70–90% response rates, but approximately 30–35% of patients discontinue the drug due to side effects such as excessive dry mouth, urinary retention, decreased sweating, skin flushing, irritability, and behavior changes [10]. Other undesirable adverse effects observed with such treatment include constipation, urinary retention, tiredness, and drowsiness [11]. Anticholinergics are contraindicated in patients with glaucoma, obstructive uropathy, gastrointestinal motility disorders, and myasthenia gravis.

Intraoral tropicamide films provide short-term relief of sialorrhea. One study provided evidence that 1 mg of tropicamide resulted in significant visual analog scale score decrease and reduction in saliva volume in nondemented PD patients [2]. Transdermal scopolamine, applied as a patch behind the ear, was well tolerated in short-term studies, but its use was limited by side effects of urinary retention and blurred vision [3].

A comprehensive systematic review of the use of anticholinergics in children concluded that benztropine, given 3–3.8 mg per day, could be effective. A significant decrease in the mean score for drooling was reported with benzhexol hydrochloride (2 × 2 up to 2 × 3 mg daily). There was also some evidence for a marked decrease in drooling with glycopyrrolate [13]. Benztropine was also reported to show a significant reduction in the total salivation scores compared to botulinum toxins A and B in a study of mixed treatment network meta-analysis of randomized controlled trials on pharmacological interventions for treating sialorrhea associated with neurological disorders [14].

Antireflux medication has also been suggested for use in drooling; however, there are no double-blind studies in the literature to offer evidence for this recommendation [2].

5.2. Botulinum toxin

The injection of botulinum toxin (BT) to the major salivary glands has grown in popularity because of its limited invasiveness and demonstrated effectiveness in many patients. It has been shown to improve quality of life of patients effectively with a low profile of side effects. However, it is important to take into account that the duration of the therapeutic effect is limited in time, generally lasting a few months [11].

The effect of BT in sialorrhea was first reported in PD patients [15]. This toxin is a potent neurotoxin that blocks the release of acetylcholine and a number of other neurotransmitters from synaptic vesicles; hence, it shows its effect by blocking cholinergic postganglionic parasympathetic fibers in sialorrhea [2].

Currently, three type A and one type B toxin are approved for use in the US. These are OnabotulinumtoxinA (BOTOX®), AbobotulinumtoxinA (Dysport®), IncobotulinumtoxinA (Xeomin®), and RimabotulinumtoxinB (Neurobloc®/myobloc®) [2]. Both A and B types of BT are reported to be effective in treatment of sialorrhea, and both have a low profile of side effects [1].

BT can be injected in parotid and/or submandibular glands. The dose, concentration, and volume of injectate, number of injections, injection site, rate of injection, gauge of needle, and distance of needle tip from the neuromuscular junction are among the factors that can affect the diffusion and spread of BT, thus its efficacy in sialorrhea. A broad dose range of BT has been reported in various studies, specifically from 10 to 100 U of Botox®, from 20 to 300 U of Dysport® per patient, while usually 2500 U of Neurobloc® per patient is reported to be injected. The effect of BT on salivation lasts for 1.5–6 months [11]. Older age is significantly associated with longer benefit duration [16]. Sometimes the reduction in salivary secretion and improvement in drooling may not be correlated, owing to the variability of the factors that influence the severity of drooling and reduction of saliva secretion [2]. Patients with PD showed a more favorable safety-efficacy ratio than did patients with ALS, due to lower adverse events and longer benefit duration [16].

In a recent meta-analysis, eight randomized placebo-controlled trials involving 181 patients were reviewed. The study reported that BT improved drooling severity in patients with sialorrhea significantly in both adult and pediatric populations. Increased saliva thickness (3.9%), dysphagia (3.3%), xerostomia (3.3%), and pneumonia (2.2%) were reported as common side effects [1]. Adverse effects such as chewing difficulties and recurrent mandibular luxation have been reported [11]. BT therapy is reported to have many advantages over other noninvasive and invasive treatments. It is effective and minimally invasive with few side effects and a low risk of aspiration. However, it is expensive and temporary, and the need for repeated sedation can be troublesome with children [2].

Ultrasound guidance for intraglandular injection is preferred by some of the authors. Blind puncture of the superficial lobe of the parotid gland following anatomical landmarks is easier, because the structure is relatively superficial. Since the submandibular glands are normally nonpalpable, infiltration may be more challenging. Ultrasound easily identifies the glandular structures for infiltration, while avoiding accidental damage to other anatomical structures, the facial nerve in the case of injection into the parotid gland, or the facial vessels in the case of the submandibular gland [11].

Jongerius et al. compared the efficacy of BT injections to transdermal scopolamine. They reported that even though both treatments were successful in significantly lowering drooling parameters, patients treated with BT did not experience any side effects, while 40% of patients taking scopolamine reported severe adverse effects. The wide range of side effects and potential drug–drug interactions encountered with scopolamine and glycopyrrolate suggests that BT may be a safer option compared to systemic anticholinergics [13].

BT can also be used for empirical selection of patients who would, in the future, be good candidates for surgical treatment of the major salivary glands. In this way, patients who respond well to BT injections can be treated more efficiently with surgery rather than receiving multiple injections. On the other hand, patients who do not respond well to BT may be considered as poor candidates for surgical treatment, because failure rates could be much higher owing to the contribution from minor salivary glands to the etiology of sialorrhea [17].

5.3. Radiation therapy

Radiation therapy to the salivary glands is a useful treatment option in elderly patients who are not candidates for surgery and cannot tolerate medications. Radiation causes xerostomia that lasts months to years. The dose may be changed to produce the desired effect, and it can be repeated if required. The main problem is that radiation can induce malignancies, but this does not happen until 10–15 years after treatment and therefore are less of a concern in patients who are elderly and debilitated [3].

5.4. Surgical treatment

While many patients are successfully treated with conservative methods and medical therapies, a number of patients are not able to tolerate the side effects of medications. BT treatment is reported to show improvement in drooling, but surgery provides a larger and longer lasting effect. Surgeons should consider more aggressive interventions for patients with chronic sialorrhea secondary to neuromuscular dysfunction with the impairment of swallowing. In these cases, sublingual or submandibular gland excision, submandibular duct ligation, parotid duct ligation, submandibular or parotid duct rerouting, or any combination of the above procedures result in higher rates of success, both short term and long term, and they may be cost-effective compared to BT injections requiring multiple visits [18]. Nevertheless, it is important to mention that surgery has a risk of permanent consequences (especially xerostomia), and that it should be preferred only in severe cases who are not responsive to nonsurgical therapies and in whom sialorrhea has great impact on the health and quality of life of the individual and caregivers [5].

Tympanic neurectomy is now regarded as a historical technique used to denervate salivary glands. This technique is performed through the middle ear, where the tympanic plexus and chorda tympani travel before entering the major salivary glands. The procedure is relatively simple and fast, but salivary function returns within 6–18 months, when nerve fibers regenerate [3, 17].

Recently, a novel procedure, transoral endoscopic submandibular ganglion neurectomy, was performed in two cases of BT-resistant drooling. Six months follow-up was successful; however, long-term results are awaiting to be warranted [19].

The most definitive treatment of sialorrhea is to excise the major salivary glands or to ligate or reroute the major salivary ducts. Surgical management can be described by a combination parotid duct ligation or rerouting with either submandibular gland excision or submandibular duct rerouting. Preservation of salivation with decrease in drooling could be accomplished by rerouting of the parotid and submandibular ducts to the posterior oropharynx with the advantage of no external scar. There may be a potential for aspiration after these procedures. Sublingual gland excision is suggested as well when the submandibular ducts are rerouted to prevent formation of salivary retention cysts. Parotid duct ligation is a simple fast procedure without an external scar, which decreases the stimulated salivary flow. There may be a risk of sialocele development. The most definitive surgical procedure, which includes bilateral parotid duct ligation and submandibular gland excision, is highly successful, with nearly total elimination of sialorrhea, a low incidence of facial weakness, and significant patient and caregiver satisfaction [3].

The meta-analysis of surgical management using a variety of surgical procedures demonstrates significant subjective relief in 81.6% of pediatric patients with sialorrhea following surgery. Bilateral submandibular gland excision and parotid duct rerouting had the highest reported success rate of 87.8%. However, simple bilateral submandibular duct rerouting and bilateral submandibular duct rerouting with bilateral parotid duct ligation had similar levels of subjective success. Four-duct ligation had the lowest success rate at 64.1%. Although this procedure seems simpler and less invasive compared to other surgeries, it can cause significant pain and swelling, since the ligated glands continue to produce saliva for a period before atrophy occurs. Bilateral submandibular duct rerouting is a procedure that is more complex than a simple submandibular duct ligation. The reported success rates with this procedure are consistently good and similar to procedures involving submandibular gland excision. Limited data suggest that fibrosis of the gland occurs due to obstruction of the rerouted duct, ending up as an actual ligation of the duct, but in most of the patients, function is maintained in at least one gland [17].

Author details

Işıl Adadan Güvenç

Address all correspondence to: isiladadan@yahoo.com

Department of Otorhinolaryngology, Head and Neck Surgery, Cigli Regional Education Hospital, Izmir, Turkey

References

[1] Vashishta R, Nguyen SA, White DR, Gillespie MB. Botulinum toxin for the treatment of sialorrhea: A meta-analysis. Otolaryngology and Head and Neck Surgery. 2013;**148**(2):191-196

[2] Lakraj AA, Moghimi N, Jabbari B. Sialorrhea: Anatomy, pathophysiology and treatment with emphasis on the role of botulinum toxins. Toxins. 2013;**5**(5):1010-1031

[3] Hockstein NG, Samadi DS, Gendron K, Handler SD. Sialorrhea: A management challenge. American Family Physician. 2004;**69**(11):2628-2634

[4] Dias BL, Fernandes AR, Maia Filho HS. Sialorrhea in children with cerebral palsy. Jornal de Pediatria. 2016;**92**(6):549-558

[5] Young CA, Ellis C, Johnson J, Sathasivam S, Pih N. Treatment for sialorrhea (excessive saliva) in people with motor neuron disease/amyotrophic lateral sclerosis. Cochrane Database of Systematic Reviews. 2011;**5**:CD006981

[6] Srivanitchapoom P, Pandey S, Hallett M. Drooling in Parkinson's disease: A review. Parkinsonism & Related Disorders. 2014;**20**(11):1109-1118

[7] Thaxter Nesbeth KA, Samuels LA, Nicholson Daley C, Gossell-Williams M, Nesbeth DA. Ptyalism in pregnancy—a review of epidemiology and practices. European Journal of Obstetrics, Gynecology, and Reproductive Biology. 2016;**198**:47-49

[8] Freudenreich O. Drug-induced sialorrhea. Drugs Today. 2005;**41**(6):411-418

[9] Bird AM, Smith TL, Walton AE. Current treatment strategies for clozapine-induced sialorrhea. The Annals of Pharmacotherapy. 2011;**45**(5):667-675

[10] Bavikatte G, Sit PL, Hassoon A. Management of drooling of saliva. British Journal of Medical Practitioners. 2012;**5**(1):a507

[11] Fuster Torres MA, Berini Aytés L, Gay Escoda C. Salivary gland application of botulinum toxin for the treatment of sialorrhea. Medicina Oral, Patología Oral y Cirugía Bucal. 2007;**12**(7):E511-E517

[12] Thomas-Stonell N, Greenberg J. Three treatment approaches and clinical factors in the reduction of drooling. Dysphagia. 1988;**3**(2):73-78

[13] Jongerius PH, van Tiel P, van Limbeek J, Gabreëls FJ, Rotteveel JJ. A systematic review for evidence of efficacy of anticholinergic drugs to treat drooling. Archives of Disease in Childhood. 2003;**88**(10):911-914

[14] Sridharan K, Sivaramakrishnan G. Pharmacological interventions for treating sialorrhea associated with neurological disorders: A mixed treatment network meta-analysis of randomized controlled trials. Journal of Clinical Neuroscience. 2018;**51**:12-17

[15] Pal PK, Calne DB, Calne S, Tsui JK. Botulinum toxin A as treatment for drooling saliva in PD. Neurology. 2000;**54**:244-247

[16] Petracca M, Guidubaldi A, Ricciardi L, Ialongo T, Del Grande A, Mulas D, et al. Botulinum toxin A and B in sialorrhea: Long-term data and literature overview. Toxicon. 2015;**107**(Pt A):129-140

[17] Reed J, Mans CK, Brietzke SE. Surgical management of drooling: A meta-analysis. Archives of Otolaryngology – Head & Neck Surgery. 2009;**135**(9):924-931

[18] Formeister EJ, Dahl JP, Rose AS. Surgical management of chronic sialorrhea in pediatric patients: 10-year experience from one tertiary care institution. International Journal of Pediatric Otorhinolaryngology. 2014;**78**(8):1387-1392

[19] Ozturk K, Erdur O, Gul O, Olmez A. Feasibility of endoscopic submandibular ganglion neurectomy for drooling. Laryngoscope. 2017;**127**(7):1604-1607

Section 2

New Approaches in the Diagnosis of Salivary Gland Diseases

Chapter 4

Salivary Diagnostics

Karolina Elżbieta Kaczor-Urbanowicz

Additional information is available at the end of the chapter

http://dx.doi.org/10.5772/intechopen.73372

Abstract

Salivary diagnostics plays an important role in the early detection and prevention of many oral and systemic diseases in a fast and noninvasive way. Saliva collection is an easy, repeatable and inexpensive diagnostic source that can be used for both diagnosis and real-time monitoring of various human diseases. In the near future, many developed and validated salivary biomarkers have the potential to reach the clinical practice. Five diagnostic "omics" constituents of saliva include proteomics, transcriptomics, metabolomics, microbiomics and microRNAs. Based on them, the newly emerging technologies of salivary diagnostics are developed that include RNA-sequencing, point-of-care technologies and liquid biopsy. They have potential to enable screening, early detection, prognosis and monitoring of various human diseases. The recent developments broadened the salivary diagnostic approach from the oral cavity to the whole physiological system, thus toward personalized individual medicine applications.

Keywords: saliva, diagnostics, oral cancer, RNA-sequencing, point-of-care, liquid biopsy

1. Introduction

Saliva is an encouraging medium to be used in the early detection, diagnosis and monitoring of oral and systemic diseases, specifically for the purpose of personalized medicine by incorporating point-of care technology platforms in the clinical settings. Though, saliva collection is easy, fast, cheap, safe, does not require specialized equipment and can be performed at home [1]. The normal daily production of saliva varies between 0.5 and 1.5 l. Saliva is an acidic biofluid, derived from the three major salivary glands (parotid, submandibular, sublingual) as well as from minor glands (labial, buccal, lingual, and palatal tissues). It is composed in vast majority of water (99%), while other constituents occur in trace amounts, including proteins and both inorganic (sodium, potassium, calcium, magnesium, chloride, etc.) and organic constituents (amylases, peroxidase, lipase, mucins, lysozyme, lactoferrins, cystatins, hormones, etc.) [2]. Salivary composition is very diverse (RNA, DNA, proteins, metabolites, and microbiota), and may be utilized for diagnostic purposes. Most importantly, salivary components may vary in their concentrations and levels depending on the individual's health or disease status. Thus, real-time monitoring of salivary data can provide useful translational clinical applications in the detection of various human oral and systemic diseases. The development of the recent technologies based on salivary diagnostics will help to introduce screening programs to enable early detection and monitoring of the disease [3].

Saliva is an important biofluid with lots of various biological functions including lubrication, chewing, swallowing, sensation, digestion and protection of oral mucosa against biological, mechanical, and chemical factors as well as infections [2].

2. Salivaomics

Currently, there are known five major diagnostic toolboxes of saliva "Salivaomics": proteomics (the study of proteins), transcriptomics (the study of RNAs), metabolomics (the study of metabolites), microRNA (the study of microRNAs) and microbiome (the study of microbiota) [1, 2] (**Figure 1**).

2.1. Proteomics

The proteomics is the large-scale screening for proteins, their expression, modifications, and interactions by using high-throughput approaches [4, 5]. Proteins can indicate various physiological and pathological states of the current health condition or specific disease. The recent advancements in proteomics contributed to the development of new non-invasive technologies.

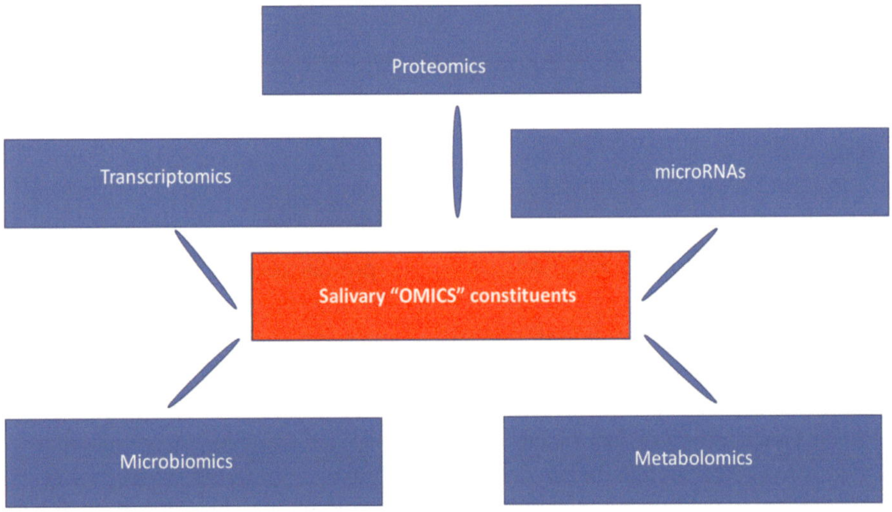

Figure 1. Diagnostic toolboxes of saliva.

The currently accepted gold standard methods for proteomic analyses include: triple depletion of high abundance proteins (removal of albumins, alpha amylase and immunoglobulins), sodium dodecyl sulfate polyacrylamide gel electrophoresis (SDS PAGE), two-dimensional gel electrophoresis (2-DE), mass spectrometry (label free qMS), ELISA (enzyme-linked immunosorbent assay) and Western blotting [2, 6]. Other advanced methods include electrospray ionization (ESI), matrix-assisted laser desorption ionization (MALDI), quadrupole/linear ion trap, time-of-flight (TOF), quadrupole TOF (QTOP), Fourier transform ion cyclotron resonance (FT-ICR), or the OrbiTrap, MS/MS, MALDI-MS or targeted HPLC-ESI-MS/MS [7].

Recently, a great focus has been put on identification of salivary protein biomarkers for various human oral and systemic diseases such as: pancreatic cancer, Sjogren's syndrome, oral cancer, lung cancer, orthodontically induced root resorption, etc. [2, 5]. The proteomics delivers an alternative ideal and non-invasive diagnostic tool, more sensitive, and safer for detecting the disease status. In addition, the depletion of high abundance proteins from saliva contributes to significant increase in the detectability of less abundant salivary proteins [5, 8]. There are known three major methods of high-abundance protein removal [9]: enzyme-substrate absorption method used for alpha-amylase affinity removal [8], immunodepletion method and combinatorial peptide ligand library (CPLL) [10].

Proteomic analysis of saliva is commonly used in the diagnostics of oral diseases as well as general health disorders such as oral candidiasis [11], oral squamous cell carcinoma (OSCC) [12], glossodynia [13], head and neck squamous cell cancer [14], Sjögren's syndrome [15], HIV [11], autism [16], fibromyalgia [17], breast cancer [18], lung cancer, melanoma [19] or pancreatic cancer [7].

Various mediators associated with oral cancer are released from cells due to malignant conditions and have been analyzed in saliva samples, like cytokines, chemokines, interferon-gamma (IFN-γ), interleukins (IL-1β, IL-6 and -8, Il-4 and -10), tumor necrosis factors (TNF-α), transforming growth factor-beta-1 (TGF-β1), epidermal growth factor (EGF), vascular endothelial growth factor (VEGF), and endothelin [20]. In case of oral squamous cell carcinoma, elevated levels of NF- κB-dependent cytokines have been observed in saliva [21]. Other potential protein biomarkers include IL-6 and S100A9 [22] or BGH3, MMP9 and PDIA3 [23]. In addition, increased salivary expression levels of MMP1 and MMP3 in OSCC patients can indicate more advanced stage of disease [12], while adenosine deaminase might be indicative of early stage of oral tongue cancer [24].

2.2. Transcriptomics

Transcriptomics (gene expression profiling) is the quantitative study of an organism's transcriptome, all RNA transcripts present in a cell. The information is recorded in the genome and expressed through transcription. These data can be used for capturing marked changes in expression levels of specific genes in the detection of various human diseases [2, 25]. Transcriptomics encompasses a great diversity of RNA species including messenger RNAs (mRNAs), long non-coding RNAs (lncRNAs), and small RNAs such as microRNAs (miRNAs), transfer RNAs (tRNAs), piwi-interacting RNA (piRNA), etc. The mRNAs play an important role in carrying information for making proteins while noncoding RNAs have different functions [25]. In turn, the microRNAs (miRNAs) are a group of small non-coding RNAs that regulate mRNA through sequence-specific binding to the UTR [26]. The miRNAs are involved in various biological processes.

The common practice in identification of salivary transcriptomic biomarkers is microarray technology. However, this technology is currently replaced by the newer one, RNA-sequencing (RNA-Seq).

2.2.1. RNA sequencing

RNA-sequencing (RNA-Seq) has been the newly developed method for characterizing the full human transcriptome. RNA-sequencing (RNA-Seq) has a wide variety of applications, but no single analysis pipeline can be used in all cases and for all biofluids [27]. Specifically, RNA-Seq of saliva is challenging, including difficult RNA isolation step to enhance yield of salivary exRNA step as well as laborious RNA-Seq small and large library construction stage, inclusion of spike in standards and controls, RNA-sequencing, data storage and data analysis. Therefore, currently available literature regarding salivary RNA-Seq is scarce [28–30].

RNA-sequencing is a rapidly progressing transcriptome profiling that uses deep-sequencing technologies and becoming the major tool in analyzing gene expression [31]. This is a new high-throughput method for both mapping and quantifying transcriptomes. It provides more detailed information about the levels of transcripts and their isoforms than other methods [32]. In general, a total RNA is converted to a library of cDNA fragments with adaptors attached to one or both ends. Afterwards, a sequencing of the molecule is performed, with or without amplification, that provides short sequences from one (single-end sequencing) or both ends (pair-end sequencing). The reads are typically 30–400 bp, depending on the DNA-sequencing technology used. Revealing the transcriptome is crucial for investigating the functional elements of the genome, the molecular constituents of cells and tissues, and also for understanding development and disease [32].

2.2.1.1. Advantages of RNA sequencing

RNA- Seq (RNA sequencing) has clear advantages over existing approaches and is believed to become the best method for analyzing transcriptome in the near future.

Firstly, RNA-Seq can be used for detection of both known (corresponding to existing genomic sequences) and novel transcripts, thus enabling identification of new organisms with unidentified yet genomic sequences. RNA-Seq is used for precise localization of transcription boundaries, to a single-base resolution. Furthermore, this method can be used for examining transcripts of great complexity as it provides useful information about the connectivity of exons as well as sequence variations in the transcribed regions [33–34].

Secondly, RNA-Seq has very low, if any, background signal. This feature differentiates it significantly from microarray platforms as it can be uniquely mapped to the genome regions of interests [35].

RNA-Seq has also significant benefits over array-based technologies for detecting expression quantitative trait loci (eQTLs). Though, it can identify different transcript variants and enable quantification of allele-specific expression within an individual to increase association mapping [27, 36, 37].

Finally, it has a highly accurate and large dynamic range of expression levels with high reproducibility rates while using less RNA sample and at a much lower cost than either tiling arrays or large-scale Sanger EST Sequencing [33, 35].

2.2.1.2. *Disadvantages of RNA sequencing*

The major problems of RNA-Seq technology are associated with RNA isolation and cDNA library construction as it includes several manipulation stages, which can complicate profiling of transcripts of various lengths [32]. This causes the variability in the measurements, influenced by the technical noise [27].

In addition, longer RNAs have to be fragmented into smaller pieces (200–500 bp) to be compatible with most deep-sequencing technologies using RNA or cDNA fragmentation methods (RNA hydrolysis or nebulization, DNase I treatment, etc.) [33, 35]. These sequencing procedures include a number of steps (RNA fragmentation, cDNA synthesis, adapter ligation, PCR amplification, bar-coding, and lane loading) that might introduce biases into the resulting data [27].

Another key consideration concerning library construction is whether or not to construct strand- specific libraries [33, 38], that provide information about the orientation of transcripts, essential for transcriptome annotation. However, strand-specific libraries are very time-consuming to produce [39, 40].

RNA-Seq has also bioinformatics challenges associated with storage, retrieval and processing large amounts of data. The alignment of long RNA-Seq reads is also complicated due to non-unique mapping to multiple locations in the genome [32].

Also, to detect a rare transcript or variant, more sequencing depth is needed. In general, the larger the genome, the more sequencing depth is required for adequate coverage, which brings greater cost [32].

Although RNA-Seq is still in the early stages of use, it has clear advantages over previously developed transcriptomic methods such as microarray profiling [32]. Specifically, salivary RNA biomarker transcripts of IL8, IL1B, DUSP1, HA3, OAZ1, S100P, and SAT yielded high sensitivity (91%) and specificity (91%) in distinguishing OSCC from the controls [41]. Also, salivary IL6 mRNA and IL-8 may serve as potential biomarkers for diagnosis of OSCC [42, 43].

2.2.2. *Difficulties in salivary RNA-sequencing and bioinformatic analysis*

RNA-sequencing (RNA Seq) of saliva is challenging compared to other biofluids such as blood or urine. RNA Sequencing of salivary samples is associated with several problems such as inadequate technique of RNA isolation, improper stabilization of RNA or RNA library construction [44–48]. Till now, there were also no established guidelines how to bioinformatically process the salivary RNA-Seq data. The recent paper by Kaczor-Urbanowicz et al. gives the recommendations for bioinformatics analysis of salivary RNA-Seq data that differs from other biofluids (blood, urine, etc.) as saliva contains the majority of microbial content, while other physiological fluids are considered to be sterile [48]. Thus, it is recommended to use quite stringent and sensitive criteria, while working with salivary RNA-Seq data to avoid erroneously mapped bacterial reads to the human genome, and to prevent problems with their further annotation to human RNA databases. In addition, the specific sequence of alignment steps and the stringency parameters associated with processing of RNA Sequencing data can grossly increase the final data quality [48].

2.3. Micro-RNA-omics

MicroRNAs (miRNAs) are short, single-stranded RNAs that are about 21 nucleotides in length. Their function is to regulate gene expression. Like other types of RNA, miRNAs are transcribed from DNA, but they do not participate in protein translation. They are non- coding RNAs, in which each primary transcript (pri-miRNA) is processed into a pre-miRNA and finally into functional miRNA [49]. Mature miRNA are involved in various biological processes such as cell growth, differentiation, apoptosis, stress and immune response or glucose secretion [50–52]. Studies on miRNA dysregulation in various human diseases have risen rapidly in recent years, including those in cancer, heart disease as well as type II diabetes mellitus and its complications, such as endothelial and vascular smooth muscle cell dysfunction, cardiomyopathy and nephropathy [53–55]. Most importantly, salivary microRNAs (miRNAs) (miR-9, miR-134 and miR-191) can be used as potential biomarkers for head and neck squamous cell carcinoma [56]. The reduction in salivary expression profiles of miR-125a and miR-200a was observed in OSCC patients compared to healthy people [57]. In turn, miR-31 increases in OSCC patients, specifically in saliva, where it rises even more than in plasma [58].

2.4. Metabolomics

Metabolomics is the study of small molecular metabolites of living tissues, mostly metabolic intermediates such as carbohydrates, lipids, amino acids, nucleic acids, etc. [1]. The major metabolomic technologies include high-performance liquid chromatography-mass spectrometry (HPLC-MS), two-dimensional gas chromatography MS and nuclear magnetic resonance spectroscopy in conjunction with pattern recognition methods [2].

Salivary metabolites are involved in many biological processes as well as pathogenesis of various diseases such as periodontal diseases, renal diseases, hepatocellular carcinoma and colorectal cancers [59] as well as oral cancer [60]. In case of oral leukoplakia, an upregulation of putrescine, 8-hydroxyadenine and 5,6-dihydrouridine in OSCC can be indicative of increased risk for malignant transformation [61].

2.5. Microbiomics

Microbiomics include study of bacteria, archaea, protists, fungi and viruses. Microbial profiling (Human Oral Microbe Identification Microarray) of salivary microbiome in early resectable pancreatic cancer revealed that Neisseria elongata and Streptococcus mitis were successfully developed with 96.4% sensitivity and 82.1% specificity [62]. Currently, newer microbiome-based technologies have been developed such as RNA or DNA sequencing [1]. In addition, two microbial biomarkers, Firmicutes (especially Streptococcus) and Actinobacteria (especially Rothia) were significantly decreased in oral cancer compared to healthy controls [63]. Finally, Furquim et al. reported that patients with Fanconi anemia (FA) are at higher risk of developing OSCC than the general population, especially after the hematopoietic stem cell transplantation [64].

3. Modern technologies in salivary diagnostics

3.1. Salivary liquid biopsy

Recently, a new trend appeared to reveal emerging role of "liquid biopsy" as identification method of biomarkers in various cancers. Liquid biopsy tests are non-invasive biofluid tests (serum, urine, saliva) that detect circulating tumor cells (CTCs) and fragments of tumor DNA shed into the bloodstream by cells undergoing apoptosis or necrosis [3].

The role of liquid biopsy markers including circulating tumor cells, circulating RNAs (miRNA, lncRNAs and mRNAs), cell-free proteins, peptides and exosomes has been currently investigated as non-invasive cancer biomarkers in different biofluids such as blood, urine, saliva and seminal plasma. Liquid biopsies hold great promise for personalized medicine due to the fact that they enable multiple non-invasive global sampling resulting in longitudinal assessment of the primary and metastatic tumors. Molecular profiling of circulating molecules (proteomic, transcriptomic, genomic, metabolomics, microRNAs) contributed to the successful application of several non-invasive multi-marker tests in the clinic [65].

Nowadays, liquid biopsy enables a variety of clinical and investigational applications such as early detection, assessment of molecular heterogeneity of general disease, monitoring of tumor dynamics (in melanoma, breast, ovarian or colon cancers), identification of genetic determinants for targeted therapy, evaluation of early treatment response, monitoring of minimal residual disease or assessment of resistance evolution in real time [66].

The most common technologies of liquid biopsy include detection and quantification of ctDNA (circulating tumor DNA) in blood such as Sanger sequencing, pyrosequencing, next generation sequencing, PCR-based technology, high-performance liquid chromatography (HPLC), mutant-enriched liquid chips, amplification refractory mutation system (ARMS), beads, emulsion, amplification and magnetics (BEAMing), pyrophosphorolysis-activated polymerization (PAP) [2, 66] or electric field-induced release and measurement (EFIRM) [67, 68]. The current gold standard methods for detection of ctDNA targets include droplet digital PCR and next-generation sequencing. However, those technologies require extraction of DNA from large volume of biofluid samples. EFIRM can be successfully used for continuous monitoring during treatment. The results are very promising [3].

Circulating tumor DNA (ctDNA) is considered to be stably found in biofluids encapsulated in extracellular vesicles (EVs) and released by cells into the circulation. If the links between distal cancers and the oral cavity will appear to be scientifically proven, it will open a new avenue of clinical utility to effectively, and non-invasively diagnose cancers through saliva. The ctDNA mutant fragments were observed in plasma [69, 70] and saliva samples [71] of head and neck cancer patients.

3.2. Point-of-care technologies

The current knowledge of salivary biomarkers and their role in point-of-care applications highlights the need for development of more advanced technologies. As a consequence, point-of-care diagnostics is definitely approaching reality for salivary research and closely related with its translation into clinical practice [3] as it delivers information of the current status of the disease in a very fast, convenient and non-invasive way. PoCs can be successfully used for early detection and real-time monitoring of the disease [3].

The current PoC technologies are ubiquitous. They comprise microfluidics, micro/nanoelectromechanical systems (MEMS/NEMS), paper-based technology, RNA-sequencing, liquid biopsy, biosensors, fluorescent biosensors, photometric and electrochemical methods, electronic nose and electric field-based methods such as electric field-induced release and measurement (EFIRM) method [3, 68, 72]. Contemporary available PoCs can be delivered in form of small and portable smartphones or "lab-on-chips" [3].

One of such PoC development is the Oral Fluid NanoSensor Test (OFNASET), that is used for multiplex detection of salivary proteomic (thioredoxin and IL-8) and genomic biomarkers (messenger RNA biomarkers, i.e. SAT, ODZ, IL-8, and IL-1b) for oral cancer with 90% sensitivity and 90% specificity for both interleukin 8 (IL-8) and IL-8 protein messenger RNA (mRNA) [67]. In turn, OraRisk human papilloma virus (HPV) test with Reflex (Quest Diagnostics, Los Angeles, CA, USA) can be indicative of HPV infection, high risk factor for development of oral cancer [68]. In addition, electrical controlled magnetic EC Sensor is designed to detect microRNA-200a [73], electrochemical sensor using endonuclease target recycling amplification to capture oral cancer overexpressed 1 (ORAOV1) [74], while wireless mouthguard enzymatic biosensor to detect uric acid [75] or lactic acid [76], potential biomarkers for oral cancer.

4. Conclusions

Salivary diagnostics is a promising field for the implementation of PoC technology. The desire for PoC, the potential of saliva, development of validated panel of salivary biomarkers for specific diseases and development of novel advanced techniques enables the application of saliva for the early detection and diagnosis of several oral and systemic diseases in a non-invasive, easy and fast personalized way. The recent technology advances, including liquid biopsy, EFIRM, biosensors, smartphones, microfluidics, paper-based technology, have the potential to make clinical utilities of saliva a reality in the near future. Saliva is predicted to be a substitute for blood, collected non-invasively for the diagnosis of oral and systemic diseases as well as chairside screening.

Acknowledgements

This work was supported by the Public Health Service (PHS) grants from the National Institute of Health (NIH): UH3 TR000923 and R90 DE022734 as well as the 2017 Debbie's Dream Foundation – American Association for Cancer Research (AACR) Gastric Cancer Research Fellowship (Grant Number 17-40-41-KACZ).

Conflict of interest

The author reports no conflict of interest in relation with the present study.

Notes/thanks/other declarations

Nothing to declare.

Author details

Karolina Elżbieta Kaczor-Urbanowicz

Address all correspondence to: kaczor.karolina@gmail.com

Department of Oral Biology and Medicine, Division of Oral Biology, UCLA Center for Oral/Head and Neck Oncology Research, UCLA Laboratory of Salivary Diagnostics, UCLA Department of Orthodontics, University of California at Los Angeles (UCLA), California, USA

References

[1] Wong DT. Salivaomics. Journal of the American Dental Association. 2012;**143**(10 Suppl): 19S-24S

[2] Kaczor-Urbanowicz KE, Martin Carreras-Presas C, Aro K, et al. Saliva diagnostics – Current views and directions. Experimantal Biology and Medicine (Maywood). 2017;**242**: 459-472. DOI: 10.1177/1535370216681550

[3] Aro K, Wei F, Wong DT, Tu M. Saliva liquid biopsy for point-of-care applications. Frontiers in Public Health. 2017;**5**:77. DOI: 10.3389/fpubh.2017.00077

[4] Anderson NL, Anderson NG. Proteome and proteomics: New technologies, new concepts, and new words. Electrophoresis. 1998;**19**:1853-1861

[5] Kaczor-Urbanowicz KE, Deutsch O, Zaks B, Krief G, Chaushu S, Palmon A. Identification of salivary protein biomarkers for orthodontically induced inflammatory root resorption. Proteomics Clinical Applications. 2017;**11**:9-10. DOI: 10.1002/prca.201600119

[6] Wong DT. Salivary diagnostics powered by nanotechnologies, proteomics and genomics. Journal of the American Dental Association (1939). 2006;**137**:313-321

[7] Lee YH, Wong DT. Saliva: An emerging biofluid for early detection of diseases. American Journal of Dentistry. 2009;**22**:241-248

[8] Deutsch O, Fleissig Y, Zaks B, Krief G, Aframian DJ, Palmon A. An approach to remove alpha amylase for proteomic analysis of low abundance biomarkers in human saliva. Electrophoresis. 2008;**29**:4150-4157. DOI: 10.1002/elps.200800207

[9] Krief G, Deutsch O, Zaks B, Wong DT, Aframian DJ, Palmon A. Comparison of diverse affinity based high-abundance protein depletion strategies for improved bio-marker discovery in oral fluids. Journal of Proteomics. 2012;**75**:4165-4175. DOI: 10.1016/j.jprot.2012.05.012

[10] Krief G, Deutsch O, Gariba S, Zaks B, Aframian DJ, Palmon A. Improved visualization of low abundance oral fluid proteins after triple depletion of alpha amylase, albumin and IgG. Oral Diseases. 2011;**17**:45-52. DOI: 10.1111/j.1601-0825.2010.01700.x

[11] Sweet SP, Denbury AN, Challacombe SJ. Salivary calprotectin levels are raised in patients with oral candidiasis or Sjogren's syndrome but decreased by HIV infection. Oral Microbiology and Immunology. 2001;**16**:119-123

[12] Stott-Miller M, Houck JR, Lohavanichbutr P, Mendez E, Upton MP, Futran ND, Schwartz SM, Chen C. Tumor and salivary matrix metalloproteinase levels are strong diagnostic markers of oral squamous cell carcinoma. Cancer Epidemiology, Biomarkers & Prevention. 2011;**20**:2628-2636. DOI: 10.1158/1055-9965.EPI-11-0503

[13] Loeb LM, Naffah-Mazzacoratti MG, Porcionatto MA, Martins JR, Kouyoumdjian M, Weckx LM, Nadera HB. Chondroitin sulfate and kallikrein in saliva: markers for glossodynia. International Immunopharmacology. 2008;**8**:1056-1058. DOI: 10.1016/j.intimp.2008.03.002

[14] Drake RR, Cazare LH, Semmes OJ, Wadsworth JT. Serum, salivary and tissue proteomics for discovery of biomarkers for head and neck cancers. Expert Review of Molecular Diagnostics. 2005;**5**:93-100. DOI: 10.1586/14737159.5.1.93

[15] Fleissig Y, Deutsch O, Reichenberg E, Redlich M, Zaks B, Palmon A, Aframian DJ. Different proteomic protein patterns in saliva of Sjogren's syndrome patients. Oral Diseases. 2009;**15**:61-68. DOI: 10.1111/j.1601-0825.2008.01465.x

[16] Castagnola M, Messana I, Inzitari R, Fanali C, Cabras T, Morelli A, Pecoraro AM, Neri G, Torrioli MG, Gurrieri F. Hypophosphorylation of salivry peptidome as a clue to the molecular pathogenesis of autism spectrum disorders. Journal of Proteome Research. 2008;**7**:5327-5332. DOI: 10.1021/pr8004088

[17] Bazzichi L, Ciregia F, Giusti L, Baldini C, Giannaccini G, Giacomelli C, Sernissi F, Bombardieri S, Lucacchini A. Detection of potential markers of primary fibromyalgia

syndrome in human saliva. Proteomics Clinical Applications. 2009;**3**:1296-1304. DOI: 10.1002/prca.200900076

[18] Streckfus CF, Bigler LR, Zwick M. The use of surface-enhanced laser desorption/ionization time-of-flight mass spectrometry to detect putative breast cancer markers in saliva: A feasibility study. Journal of Oral Pathology & Medicine. 2006;**35**:292-300. DOI: 10.1111/j.1600-0714.2006.00427.x

[19] Gao K, Zhou H, Zhang L, Lee JW, Zhou Q, Hu S, Wolinsky LE, Farrell J, Eibl G, Wong DT. Systemic disease-induced salivary biomarker profiles in mouse models of melanoma and non-small cell lung cancer. PLoS One. 2009;**4**:e5875. DOI: 10.1371/journal.pone.0005875

[20] Prasad G, McCullough M. Chemokines and cytokines as salivary biomarkers for the early diagnosis of oral cancer. International Journal of Dentistry. 2013;**2013**:813756. DOI: 10.1155/2013/813756

[21] Rhodus NL, Cheng B, Myers S, Miller L, Ho V, Ondrey F. The feasibility of monitoring NF-kappaB associated cytokines: TNF-alpha, IL-1alpha, IL-6, and IL-8 in whole saliva for the malignant transformation of oral lichen planus. Molecular Carcinogenesis. 2005;**44**:77-82. DOI: 10.1002/mc.20113

[22] Csosz E, Labiscsak P, Kallo G, Markus B, Emri M, Szabo A, et al. Proteomics investigation of OSCC-specific salivary biomarkers in a Hungarian population highlights the importance of identification of population-tailored biomarkers. PLoS One. 2017;**12**:e0177282. DOI: 10.1371/journal.pone.0177282

[23] He Y, Shao F, Pi W, Shi C, Chen Y, Gong D, et al. Largescale transcriptomics analysis suggests over-expression of BGH3, MMP9 and PDIA3 in oral squamous cell carcinoma. PLoS One. 2016;**11**:e0146530. DOI: 10.1371/journal.pone.0146530

[24] Rai B, Kaur J, Jacobs R, Anand SC. Adenosine deaminase in saliva as a diagnostic marker of squamous cell carcinoma of tongue. Clinical Oral Investigations. 2011;**15**:347-349. DOI: 10.1007/s00784-010-0404-z

[25] Lowe R, Shirley N, Bleackley M, et al. Transcriptomics technologies. PLoS. Computational Biology. 2017;**13**:e1005457. DOI: 10.1371/journal.pcbi.1005457

[26] He L, Hannon GE. MicroRNAs: Small RNAs with a big role in gene regulation. Nature Reviews. Genetics. 2004;**5**:522-531. DOI: 10.1038/nrg1379

[27] Conesa A, Madrigal P, Tarazona S, Gomez-Cabrero D, Cervera A, McPherson A, Szcześniak MW, Gaffney DJ, Elo LL, Zhang X, Mortazavi A. A survey of best practices for RNA-seq data analysis. Genome Biology. 2016;**17**:13. DOI: 10.1186/s13059-016-0881-8

[28] Takeshita T, Kageyama S, Furuta M, Tsuboi H, Takeuchi K, Shibata Y, Shimazaki Y, Akifusa S, Ninomiya T, Kiyohara Y, Yamashita Y. Bacterial diversity in saliva and oral health-related conditions: The Hisayama study. Scientific Reports. 2016;**6**:22164. DOI: 10.1038/srep22164

[29] Yeri A, Courtright A, Reiman R, Carlson E, Beecroft T, Janss A, Siniard A, Richholt R, Balak C, Rozowsky J, Kitchen R, Hutchins E, Winarta J, McCoy R, Anastasi M, Kim S,

Huentelman M, Van Keuren-Jensen K. Total extracellular small RNA profiles from plasma, saliva, and urine of healthy subjects. Scientific Reports. 2017;**7**:44061. DOI: 10.1038/srep44061

[30] Majem B, Li F, Sun J, Wong DT. RNA sequencing analysis of salivary extracellular RNA. Methods in Molecular Biology. 2017;**1537**:17-36. DOI: 10.1007/978-1-4939-6685-1_2

[31] Choy JY, Boon PL, Bertin N, Fullwood MJ. A resource of ribosomal RNA-depleted RNA-Seq data from different normal adult and fetal human tissues. Scientific Data. 2015;**2**: 150063. DOI: 10.1038/sdata.2015.63

[32] Wang Z, Gerstein M, Snyder M. RNA-Seq: A revolutionary tool for transcriptomics. Nature Reviews. Genetics. 2009;**10**:57-63. DOI: 10.1038/nrg2484

[33] Cloonan N, Forrest AR, Kolle G, et al. Stem cell transcriptome profiling via massive-scale mRNA sequencing. Nature Methods. 2008;**5**:613-619. DOI: 10.1038/nmeth.1223

[34] Morin R, Bainbridge M, Fejers A, et al. Profiling the HeLa S3 transcriptome using randomly primed cDNA and massively parallel short-read sequencing. BioTechniques. 2008;**45**:81-94. DOI: 10.2144/000112900

[35] Mortazavi A, Williams BA, McCue K, Schaeffer L, Wold B. Mapping and quantifying mammalian transcriptomes by RNA-Seq. Nature Methods. 2008;**5**:621-628. DOI: 10.1038/nmeth.1226

[36] Kumasaka N, Knights AJ, Gaffney DJ. Fine-mapping cellular QTLs with RASQUAL and ATAC-seq. Nature Genetics. 2016;**48**:206-213. DOI: 10.1038/ng.3467

[37] Nagalakshmi U, Wang Z, Waern K et al. The transcriptional landscape of the yeast genome defined by RNA sequencing. Science. 2008;**320**:1344-1349. DOI: 10.1126/science.1158441

[38] Lister R, O'Malley RC, Tonti-Filippini J, Gregory BD, Berry CC, Millar AH, Ecker JR. Highly integrated single-base resolution maps of the epigenome in Arabidopsis. Cell. 2008;**133**:523-536. DOI: 10.1016/j.cell.2008.03.029

[39] Wilhelm BT, Marguerat S, Watt S, Schubert F, Wood V, Goodhead I, Penkett CJ, Rogers J, Bähler J. Dynamic repertoire of a eukaryotic transcriptome surveyed at single-nucleotide resolution. Nature. 2008;**453**:1239-1243. DOI: 10.1038/nature07002

[40] Dutrow N, Nix DA, Holt D, Milash B, Dalley B, Westbroek E, Parnell TJ, Cairns BR. Dynamic transcriptome of schizosaccharomyces pombe shown by RNA-DNA hybrid mapping. Nature Genetics. 2008;**40**:977-986. DOI: 10.1038/ng.196

[41] Li Y, St John MA, Zhou X, Kim Y, Sinha U, Jordan RC, et al. Salivary transcriptome diagnostics for oral cancer detection. Clinical Cancer Research. 2004;**10**:8442-8450. DOI: 10.1158/1078-0432.CCR-04-1167

[42] Horvath J, Szabo A, Tar I, Dezso B, Kiss C, Marton I, et al. Oral health may affect the performance of mRNA-based saliva biomarkers for oral squamous cell cancer. Pathology Oncology Research. 2017. [Epub ahead of print]. DOI: 10.1007/s12253-017-0296-1

[43] Khyani IAM, Qureshi MA, Mirza T, Farooq MU. Detection of interleukins-6 and 8 in saliva as potential biomarkers of oral pre-malignant lesion and oral carcinoma: A breakthrough in salivary diagnostics in Pakistan. Pakistan Journal of Pharmaceutical Sciences. 2017;**30**:817-823

[44] Spielmann N, Ilsley D, Gu J, Lea K, Brockman J, Heater S, Setterquist R, Wong DT. The human salivary RNA transcriptome revealed by massively parallel sequencing. Clinical Chemistry. 2012;**58**:1314-1321. DOI: 10.1373/clinchem.2011.176941

[45] Burgos KL, Javaherian A, Bomprezzi R, Ghaffari L, Rhodes S, Courtright A, Tembe W, Kim S, Metpally R, Van Keuren-Jensen K. Identification of extracellular miRNA in human cerebrospinal fluid by next-generation sequencing. Ribonucleic Acid. 2013;**19**:712-722. DOI: 10.1261/rna.036863.112

[46] Hu L, Wu C, Guo C, Li H, Xiong C. Identification of microRNAs predominately derived from testis and epididymis in human seminal plasma. Clinical Biochemistry. 2014;**47**: 967-972

[47] Bahn JH, Zhang Q, Li F, Chan TM, Lin X, Kim Y, Wong DT, Xiao X. The landscape of microRNA, piwi-interacting RNA, and circular RNA in human saliva. Clinical Chemistry. 2015;**61**:221-230. DOI: 10.1016/j.clinbiochem.2013.11.009

[48] Kaczor-Urbanowicz KE, Kim Y, Li F, Galeev T, Kitchen RR, Koyano K, Jeong SH, Wang X, Elashoff D, Kang SY, Kim SM, Kim K, Kim S, Chia D, Xiao X, Rozowsky J, Wong DTW. Novel approaches for bioinformatic analysis of salivary RNA sequencing data in the biomarker development process. Bioinformatics. 2017. [Epub ahead of print]. DOI: 10.1093/bioinformatics/btx504

[49] Macfarlane LA, Murphy PR. MicroRNA: Biogenesis, function and role in cancer. Current Genomics. 2010;**11**:537-561. DOI: 10.2174/138920210793175895

[50] Lu J, Getz G, Miska EA, Alvarez-Saavedra E, Lamb J, Peck D, Sweet-Cordero A, Ebert BL, Mak RH, Ferrando AA, Downing JR, Jacks T, Horvitz HR, Golub TR. MicroRNA expression profiles classify human cancers. Nature. 2005;**435**:834-838. DOI: 10.1038/nature03702

[51] Stadler BM, Ruohola-Baker H. Small RNAs: Keeping stem cells in line. Cell. 2008;**132**:563-566. DOI: 10.1016/j.cell.2008.02.005

[52] Taganov KD, Boldin MP, Baltimore D. MicroRNAs and immunity: Tiny players in a big field. Immunity. 2007;**26**:133-137. DOI: 10.1016/j.immuni.2007.02.005

[53] Zitman-Gal T, Green J, Pasmanik-Chor M, et al. Vitamin D manipulates miR-181c, miR-20b and miR-15a in human umbilical vein endothelial cells exposed to a diabetic-like environment. Cardiovascular Diabetology 2014;**13**:8. DOI: 10.1186/1475-2840-13-8

[54] Lorenzen J, Kumarswamy R, Dangwal S, Thum T. MicroRN in diabetes and diabetes-associated complications. RNA Biology. 2012;**9**:820-827. DOI: 10.4161/rna.20162

[55] Caporali A, Meloni M, Völlenkle C, et al. Deregulation of microRNA-503 contributes to diabetes mellitus-induced impairment of endothelial function and reparative angiogenesis

after limb ischemia. Circulation. 2011;**123**:282-291. DOI: 10.1161/CIRCULATIONAHA.110.952325

[56] Salazar C, Nagadia R, Pandit P, Cooper-White J, Banerjee N, et al. A novel saliva-based microRNA biomarker panel to detect head and neck cancers. Cellular Oncology. 2014;**37**:331-338. DOI: 10.1007/s13402-014-0188-2

[57] Park NJ, Zhou H, Elashoff D, Henson BS, Kastratovic DA, Abemayor E, et al. Salivary microRNA: Discovery, characterization, and clinical utility for oral cancer detection. Clinical Cancer Research. 2009;**15**:5473-5477. DOI: 10.1158/1078-0432.CCR-09-0736

[58] Liu CJ, Lin SC, Yang CC, Cheng HW, Chang KW. Exploiting salivary miR-31 as a clinical biomarker of oral squamous cell carcinoma. Head & Neck. 2012;**34**:219-224. DOI: 10.1002/hed.21713

[59] Beger RD. A review of applications of metabolomics in cancer. Metabolites. 2013;**3**:552-574. DOI: 10.3390/metabo3030552

[60] Mikkonen JJ, Singh SP, Herrala M, Lappalainen R, Myllymaa S, Kullaa AM. Salivary metabolomics in the diagnosis of oral cancer and periodontal diseases. Journal of Periodontal Research. 2016;**51**:431-437. DOI: 10.1111/jre.12327

[61] Sridharan G, Ramani P, Patankar S. Serum metabolomics in oral leukoplakia and oral squamous cell carcinoma. Journal of Cancer Research and Therapeutics. 2017;**13**:556-561. DOI: 10.4103/jcrt.JCRT_1233_16

[62] Farrell JJ, Zhang L, Zhou H, Chia D, Elashoff D, Akin D, Paster BJ, Joshipura K, Wong DT. Variations of oral microbiota are associated with pancreatic diseases including pancreatic cancer. Gut. 2012;**61**:582-588. DOI: 10.1136/gutjnl-2011-300784

[63] Schmidt BL, Kuczynski J, Bhattacharya A, Huey B, Corby PM, Queiroz EL, et al. Changes in abundance of oral microbiota associated with oral cancer. PLoS One. 2014;**9**:e98741. DOI: 10.1371/journal.pone.0098741

[64] Furquim CP, Soares GM, Ribeiro LL, Azcarate-Peril MA, Butz N, Roach J, et al. The salivary microbiome and oral cancer risk: A pilot study in fanconi anemia. Journal of Dental Research. 2017;**96**:292-299. DOI: 10.1177/0022034516678169

[65] Di Meo A, Bartlett J, Cheng Y, Pasic MD, Yousef GM. Liquid biopsy: A step forward towards precision medicine in urologic malignancies. Molecular Cancer. 2017;**16**:80. DOI: 10.1186/s12943-017-0644-5

[66] Diaz Jr, LA, Bardelli A. Liquid biopsies: Genotyping circulating tumor DNA. Journal of Clinical Oncology 2014;**32**:579-586. DOI: 10.1200/JCO.2012.45.2011

[67] Wei F, Lin CC, Joon A, Feng Z, Troche G, Lira ME, Chia D, Mao M, Ho CL, Su WC, Wong DT. Noninvasive saliva-based EGFR gene mutation detection in patients with lung cancer. American Journal of Respiratory and Critical Care Medicine. 2014;**190**:1117-1126. DOI: 10.1164/rccm.201406-1003OC

[68] Kaczor-Urbanowicz KE, Martín Carreras-Presas C, Kaczor T, Tu M, Wei F, Garcia-Godoy F, Wong DT. Emerging technologies for salivaomics in cancer detection. Journal of Cellular and Molecular Medicine. 2017;**21**:640-647. DOI: 10.1111/jcmm.13007

[69] Bettegowda C, Sausen M, Leary RJ, Kinde I, Wang Y, Agrawal N, et al. Detection of circulating tumor DNA in early- and late-stage human malignancies. Science Translational Medicine. 2014;**6**:224ra24. DOI: 10.1126/scitranslmed.3007094

[70] Lebofsky R, Decraene C, Bernard V, Kamal M, Blin A, Leroy Q, et al. Circulating tumor DNA as a non-invasive substitute to metastasis biopsy for tumor genotyping and personalized medicine in a prospective trial across all tumor types. Molecular Oncology. 2015;**9**:783-790. DOI: 10.1016/j.molonc.2014.12.003

[71] Wang Y, Springer S, Mulvey CL, Silliman N, Schaefer J, Sausen M, et al. Detection of somatic mutations and HPV in the saliva and plasma of patients with head and neck squamous cell carcinomas. Science Translational Medicine. 2015;**7**:293ra104. DOI: 10.1126/scitranslmed.aaa8507

[72] Khan RS, Khurshid Z, Asiri FYI. Advancing point-of-care (PoC) testing using human saliva as liquid biopsy. Diagnostics (Basel). 2017;**7**:39. DOI: 10.3390/diagnostics7030039

[73] Wang Z, Zhang J, Guo Y, et al. A novel electrically magnetic-controllable electrochemical biosensor for the ultrasensitive and specific detection of attomolar level oral cancer-related microRNA. Biosensors & Bioelectronics. 2013;**45**:108-113. DOI: 10.1016/j.bios.2013.02.007

[74] Tan Y, Wei X, Zhao M, et al. Ultraselective homogeneous electrochemical biosensor for DNA species related to oral cancer based on nicking endonuclease assisted target recycling amplification. Analytical Chemistry. 2015;**87**:9204-9208. DOI: 10.1021/acs.analchem.5b01470

[75] Kim J, Vald es-Ram ırez G, Bandodkar AJ, et al. Non-invasive mouthguard biosensor for continuous salivary monitoring of metabolites. The Analyst 2014;**139**:1632-1666. DOI: 10.1039/c3an02359a

[76] Kim J, Imani S, de Araujo WR, et al. Wearable salivary uric acid mouthguard biosensor with integrated wireless electronics. Biosensors & Bioelectronics 2015;**74**:1061-1068. DOI: 10.1016/j.bios.2015.07.039

Chapter 5

Proteomics of the Salivary Fluid

Goran Mitulović

Additional information is available at the end of the chapter

http://dx.doi.org/10.5772/intechopen.72309

Abstract

Following the sequencing of the human genome, the mapping of the human proteome is the next task to being completed in order to gain knowledge on how proteins are involved in disease genesis, growth, therapy, and healing. As contrary to the genome, which is relatively static, the human proteome is significantly more complex and highly dynamic. Whilst the majority of the research is being focused on analyzing either the proteome of tumor tissues and tumor cells or the proteome of serum and plasma, little attention has been awarded to the analysis of proteomes in saliva or urine. The proteome in saliva can help providing important information on processes involving health issues in dentistry, head and neck cancers, gastric cancers or neurology, to name just a few. However, this is changing and the proteomics research community is increasingly focusing on deciphering the salivary proteome. So far, more than 3000 proteins have been identified in different studies and more is to come with new instrumentation and methods available. Some of the proteomics methods applied for analysis of salivary proteins will be discussed in this chapter.

Keywords: salival, proteomics, diagnostics, biomarkers, chromatography, mass spectrometry

1. Introduction

The raise of proteomics and the continuous development and improvement of analytical instruments such as high-performance liquid chromatography (HPLC) and mass spectrometry (MS) have substantially fuelled the development of instrumental methods for analysis of proteins for both research and clinical questions [1–6]. Proteomics is not only addressing the efficient separation of peptides upon, mostly, tryptic digestion of proteins and their sensitive detection using mass spectrometry. Proteomics is a technology enabling significantly and profoundly better approach to investigating and understanding proteins' function and their posttranslational modifications [7–12]. Applying proteomics methods for analysis of clinical samples is especially important in time of personalized medicine, which tailors individualized treatment of each patient based on specification of the diseases [3, 13–19]. Furthermore, (clinical) proteomics can be used as a method-of-choice for the screening of biomarkers used for early discovery and early diagnostics. Early diagnostics and early discovery, needless to say, will help decreasing patients' morbidity and mortality by detecting the disease at the stage when it can be effectively treated with less side effects and at significantly lower cost for the society. This approach can be very beneficial especially for diseases affecting large populations such as cardiovascular diseases, diabetes mellitus and other endocrinal diseases, glioblastoma and similar.

Proteomics can also be applied for the point-of-care diagnostic approaches where both medical professionals and patients can get rapid information and bed-side diagnosis. Of course, classic proteomics approaches with protein extraction from tissue or body fluids and overnight protein digestion cannot be applied; however, proteomics can provide information to be used with kits for point-of-care approach [20–24].

It has already been shown that saliva is a highly valid biological fluid that can be used for diagnostic applications [25–39].

Various number of components can be identified in saliva, which provides real-time data on the patient's condition. The substances found in saliva include but are not limited to DNA, RNA, proteins, metabolites, and microbiota from both oral and gastrointestinal origin. Sample collection is simple, cheap, and can be provided by patient at home without expensive equipment or medical personal needed on-site.

This manuscript will provide a short insight into different techniques applied for proteomics analysis of saliva starting with sample collection, protein precipitation and digestion, peptide separation and MS detection, and finally with data analysis.

2. Sample collection

For medical or biological analysis in general, the method how and when a sample is being collected is of utmost importance. Sample collection is one of the pre-analytical steps that need extraordinary caution and that can influence, badly in most cases, the complete process of sample analysis.

Saliva is mainly composed of water; however, there are a number of other substances being present. Mucins, proteins, DNA, RNA, enzymes, sugars, cell debris, and microbiota and their secretome can interfere with test performance. Therefore, an optimized sample collection process is needed, and a researcher must carefully and cautiously prepare the sample collection step, and the patient must be educated and trained if sample is being to be collected at home. Furthermore, steps like sample storage and transport to the laboratory must also be carefully planned and executed especially when longitudinal studies of the same patient or of the patients' groups are being performed, and especially in parts of the world where appropriate infrastructure is not always available [40–45].

Several methods can be applied for collection of saliva: (1) passive droll is the simplest approach but the saliva often has a high concentration of mucins and high viscosity and (2) the Salivette® Systems [46–48], the Greiner Bio-One Saliva Kit, and the recently introduced

RNA-Prosal [49]. All three sample collection systems have been used in the field, and publications describing their efficacy are available [50–52].

At the Proteomics Core Facility of the Medical University of Vienna Salivette® is being used for induced saliva sample collection by chewing cotton swabs. As mentioned previously, it is of great importance to carefully plan and perform sample collection. The patient or the donor must retain from consuming food, alcoholic beverage, and caffeine at least for 2 h before sample collection. Further, the patient shall briefly wash the mouth using water only. Saliva is being collected for 2 min during which the patient chews the cotton swab. This approach yields approximately 2.5 ml of saliva, which is sufficient for performing proteomics analysis. Some patients, however, need additional stimulation for saliva production and paraffin gum can be used in these cases to stimulate saliva flow and gain enough sample volume. In these cases, the use of Greiner Bio-One Kit helps obtaining more saliva than chewing the cotton swab; however, one shall be careful since this kit contains citric acid, which can lead to protein denaturation and protein loss during the sample collection.

As soon as the sample has been collected it shall be supplemented with enzyme inhibitors in order to suppress enzyme activity and protein degradation. A total protease inhibitor cocktail such as Roche's "Complete Protease Inhibitor Cocktail®" is being added to the sample following centrifugation and removal of cellular debris and prior to storage at −80°C.

It is of extreme importance to secure reproducible sample collection procedures and properly train the patients in cases of self-sampling to avoid sample contamination and alteration. Furthermore, conditions for proper sample transportation and handling until it is being processed must also be carefully considered and applied.

Table 1 shows the steps applied for sample collection and the preparative work.

Step	Device	Temperature	Precautions
1. Sample collection	Salivette® (used in the Proteomics Core Facility at the Medical University in Vienna)	Human body	No food, alcoholic or caffeine beverages until 2 h before sample collection!
2. Centrifugation	Centrifuge	4°C	
3. Protein precipitation	Modified Wessel-Fluegge as described or Aceton	According to the protocol described	Sample should always be prepared on ice!
4. Depletion of high abundant proteins	Antihuman serum albumin and Anti-IgG columns and anti-amylase column	Ambient to 40°C	Pay attention to columns' loadability!
5. Enzymatic digest	Offline digest overnight	37°C	
6. (Multidimensional) HPLC separation and MS detection of tryptic peptides	Nano HPLC and mass spectrometer	Various combinations	Column capacity, compatibility of selected separation dimensions
7. Bioinformatics-Database search	Various platforms are available	Not relevant	Carefully select parameters, avoid very stringent but also very lax conditions
8. Verification and Validation			

Table 1. General description of sample preparation for proteomics analysis of salivary samples.

3. Sample preparation: depletion of abundant proteins and enzymatic digest

The enzymatic digest of salivary proteins does not differ from digestion of other proteins. Usually, trypsin is being used for proteolytic cleavage of proteins due to its relatively high specificity, availability, and ease of use. Furthermore, tryptic peptides are ideally suited for reversed phase HPLC separation and positive ionization using electrospray MS (ESI). Tryptic peptides are also ideal for using multidimensional separation approaches such as strong cation exchange (SCX), hydrophilic interaction liquid chromatography (HILIC), or electrostatic repulsion interaction chromatography (ERLIC) since they bear positive charges on N-terminus or Lys-residues.

Beside trypsin, other proteases can also be used alone or in combination with trypsin. The aim is either to achieve specific cleavage of proteins for special questions or to achieve smaller peptides and enhance their ionization, detection, and ultimately better sequence coverage for identified proteins. Mostly, proteins such as Lys-C and GluC are applied for pre-digestion before trypsin addition.

Protein digest begins with protein precipitation from saliva. A number of methods have been developed for protein precipitation such as: (1) alcoholic; (2) salting out; (3) applying strong acids (trichloroacetic acid); (4) using acetone; (5) using acetonitrile, etc. Protein precipitation shall help for removing DNA and RNA and their fragments from the sample and for removing lipids.

The Proteomics Core Facility of the Medical University in Vienna applies a modified Wessel-Fluegge [53] method for protein precipitation [54]. **Figure 1** shows the sample collection steps prior to protein reduction, alkylation, and addition of the protease.

In addition to trypsin, the use of proteases, e.g. LysC, will help generating smaller peptides prior to separation and detection [55, 56].

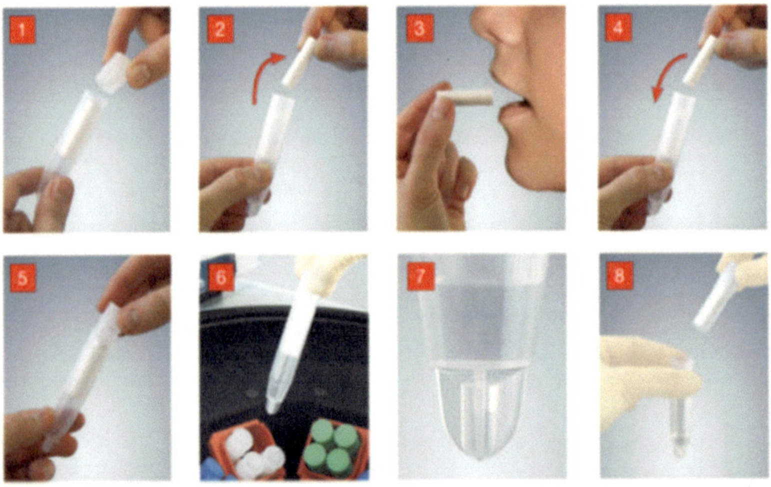

Figure 1. Sample collection steps prior to protein reduction, alkylation, and addition of the protease as performed at the Proteomics Core Facility of the Medical University of Vienna (https://www.sarstedt.com/en/products/diagnostic/salivasputum/product/51.1534.500/).

http://dx.doi.org/10.5772/intechopen.72309

Unlike serum or plasma, saliva does not contain large range and amounts of high abundant proteins such as serum albumin or hemoglobin that can affect sensitivity and selectivity of detection. However, amylase and serum albumin are still proteins with the highest abundance in saliva and can also affect the detection of other low abundant species and should be removed from the sample [57, 58]. In human saliva, alpha-amylase makes about 60% of the abundance of all proteins present, and its removal will help identifying proteins of lower abundance such as cytokines, which can be used as putative biomarkers for different processes. Deutsch et al. [57] have shown a simple yet very effective method for removing alpha-amylase and gaining a deeper insight into saliva's proteome. The use of a simple potato starch resulted in sixfold reduction of the amount of alpha-amylase in the sample. Albumin removal can be facilitated by using a number of columns developed and based on immunoaffinity reactions [59].

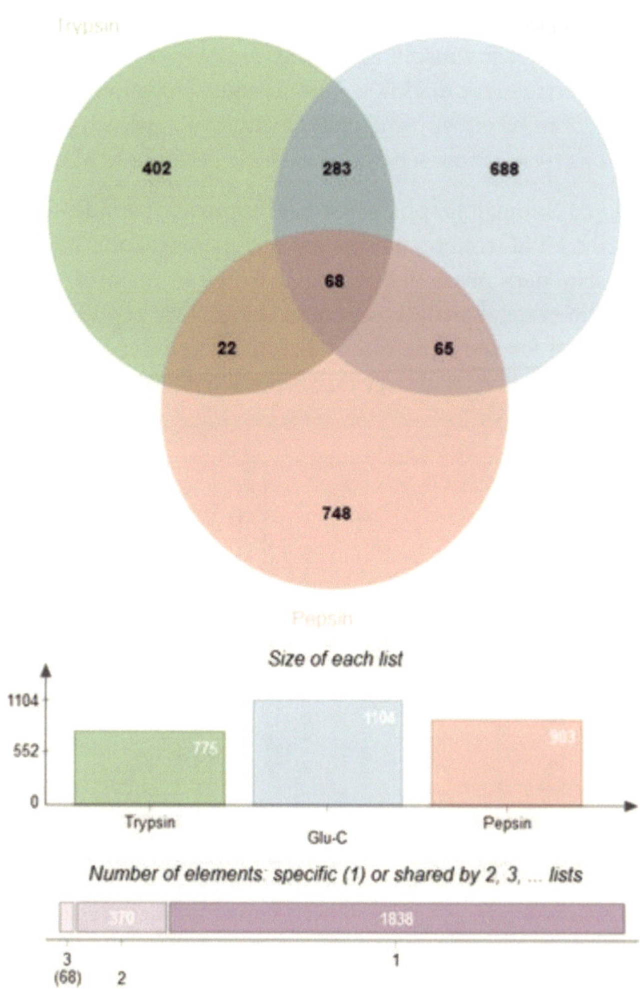

Figure 2. Comparison of the number of identified proteins from human saliva by applying different proteases. Courtesy of Zofia Świątczak (Master Thesis).

Enzymatic digest of salivary proteins does not differ from enzymatic digests used for other biological samples. Based on previous experience and results, trypsin is the most widely used protease for protein digest resulting with peptides suited for subsequent separation using cation exchange columns or anion exchange columns, reversed phase separation, and mass spectrometric detection. A comparison of results obtained using different digestion methods for salivary samples obtained from healthy donors is shown in **Figure 2**.

As shown, the highest number of proteins was identified upon applying a combined digestion approach and using GluC and trypsin. However, the choice of proteases used also depends on analytical problem to be addressed as, e.g. for detection of glycosylated proteins, which might require additional proteases to be applied.

4. Chromatographic separation of digested proteins

Upon tryptic digestion of proteins, resulting peptides are being separated on a chromatographic column prior to mass spectrometric detection and subsequent bioinformatics analysis. Separation of peptides is being performed either using one-dimensional approach or the multidimensional separation by combining two or more separation technologies prior to MS detection and analysis.

For the one-dimensional chromatographic separation approach, peptides are being injected onto the reversed phase nano HPLC column where they are separated according to their hydrophobic interaction with the stationary phase [60]. **Figure 2** shows an exemplary base peak chromatogram (BPC) for one-dimensional analysis separation of salivary peptides. Usually, long separation gradients are selected for one-dimensional separation in order to provide the best possible conditions for peptide separations and large number of identifications.

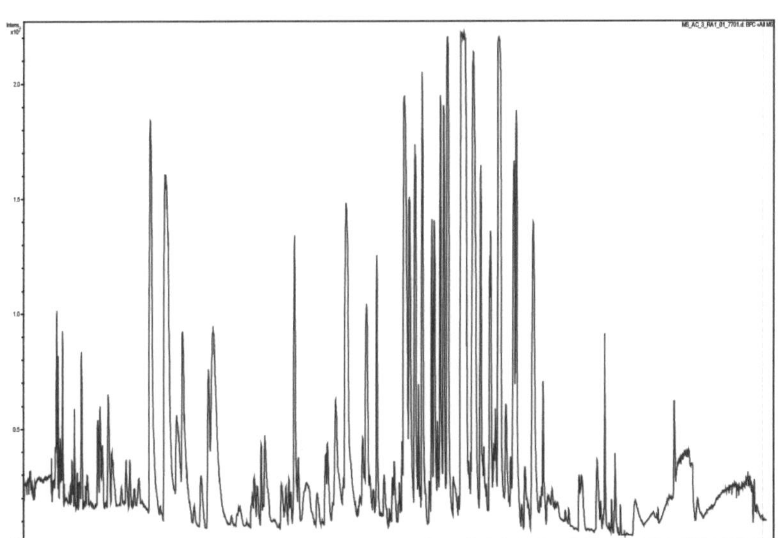

Figure 3. Base Peak Chromatogram (BPC) of GluC-tryptically generated peptides, which were separated on a reversed phase nano HPLC column.

The separation shown in **Figure 3** was performed using a 180-min gradient and a total analysis runtime of 210 min. Thus, the total amount of available time must be considered when performing this kind of analysis.

The use of multidimensional separation methods will increase the number of peptides detected and the number of identified proteins, and, in addition, protein's sequence coverage will be

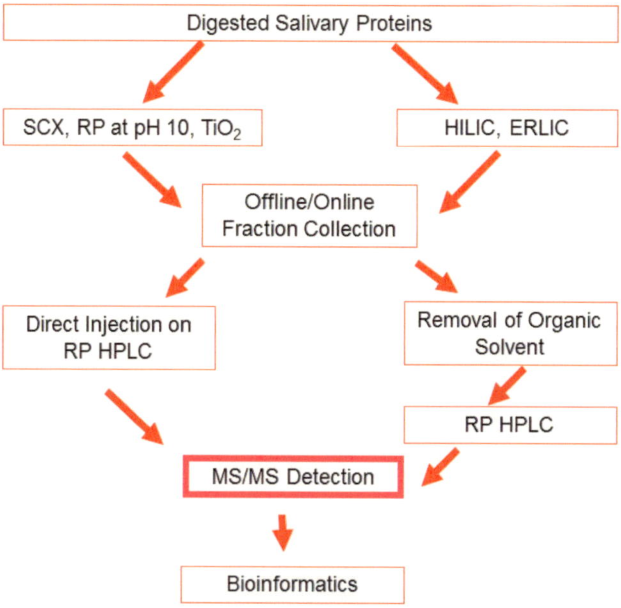

Figure 4. A number of combinations of different techniques can be used for separation of peptides and proteins in a proteomics approach.

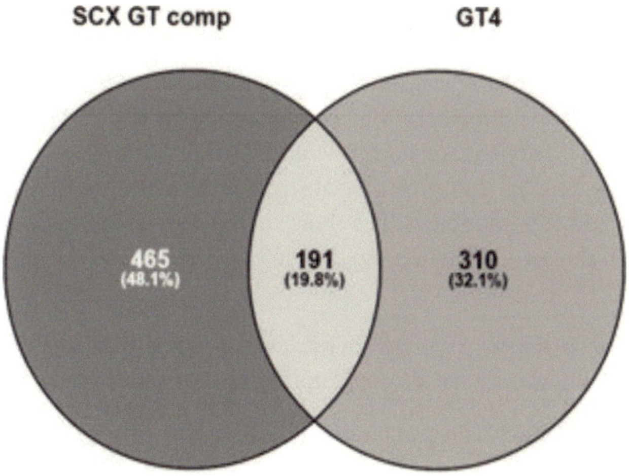

Figure 5. Two-dimensional separation approach for salivary peptides enables identification of higher number of proteins. Data courtesy of Zofia Świątczak (Master Thesis).

improved for identified proteins. Improved sequence coverage for identified proteins is one of the major challenges for proteomics analysis with high importance since it enhances chances for detection of posttranslational modifications (PTM) such as phosphorylation, glycosylation, methylation, etc., which are important as drug targets.

Different types of separation approaches can be used for the two-dimensional approach: strong cation exchange columns, weak anion exchange columns, reversed phase columns at high pH, and other combinations are possible [61–63]. A schematic of possible combinations of chromatographic approaches is shown in **Figure 4**.

Generally, the use of multidimensional separation will result in increased number of identifications, and **Figure 5** shows the comparison of the number of detected proteins upon applying the two-dimensional chromatographic separation with strong cation exchange column used for the first separation dimension.

5. Mass spectrometric detection and bioinformatics analysis

Upon separation, peptides are being detected using mass spectrometry and analyzed by comparing experimental data and databases of in-silico digested proteins. Several MS approaches have been applied for detection of salivary peptides: Electrospray Time-of-Flight (ESI-ToF), MALDI-Time-of-Flight (MALDI-ToF), ESI-Orbitrap analysis, ESI-Quadrupole ToF, etc.

Depending on MS type and selected instrumental method, posttranslational modifications of proteins can also be identified and thoroughly analyzed thus enabled a deeper insight into the proteome. The majority of top-down analysis, i.e. analysis of undigested proteins is performed using MALDI mass spectrometers, and the majority of analysis for digested proteins (peptides) is performed using electrospray (ESI) ionization and ToF and Orbitrap mass analyzer.

The analysis of obtained raw data is performed by searching protein databases such as SwissProt, Uniprot, NR (by NCBI), and user-generated databases. A number of commercially available software packages such as Mascot (Matrix Science, London), ProteinScape (Bruker, Germany), Proteome Discoverer (Thermo Scientific, Bremen, Germany), and of free available software such as The Global Proteome Machine (www.thegpm.org), MaxQuant (http://www.coxdocs.org/doku.php?id=maxquant:start), PeptideShaker (http://www.uib.no/en/rg/probe/65218/peptideshaker), Skyline (https://skyline.ms/project/home/begin.view?), OpenMS (https://www.openms.de/), and other packages. The choice of the software to be used strongly depends not only on personal preferences but also on data to be analyzed and the information needed to be extracted.

Figure 6 shows a screenshot of two software packages preferably used at the Proteomics Core Facility at the Medical University of Vienna, Peptide Shaker and ProteinScape.

In addition to database search and protein identification, the analysis of the pathways where proteins are being over- or underexpressed and the analysis of interactions with other proteins have been performed using free software such as DAVID® (https://david.ncifcrf.gov/), STRING (https://string-db.org/), Reactome (http://reactome.org/) or commercially available MetaCore® (http://lsresearch.thomsonreuters.com/) or similar.

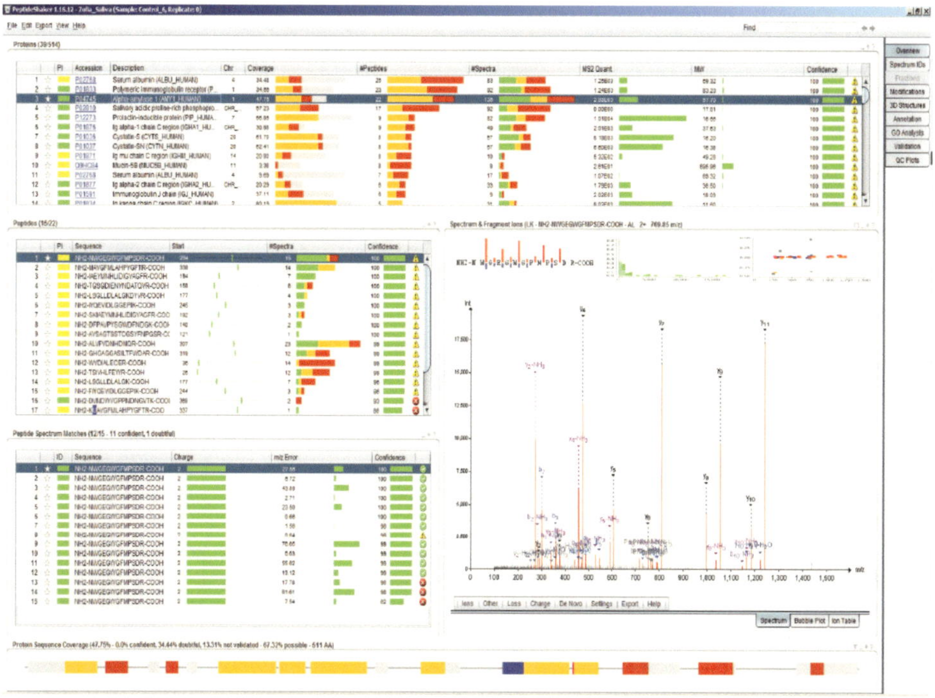

Peptide Shaker

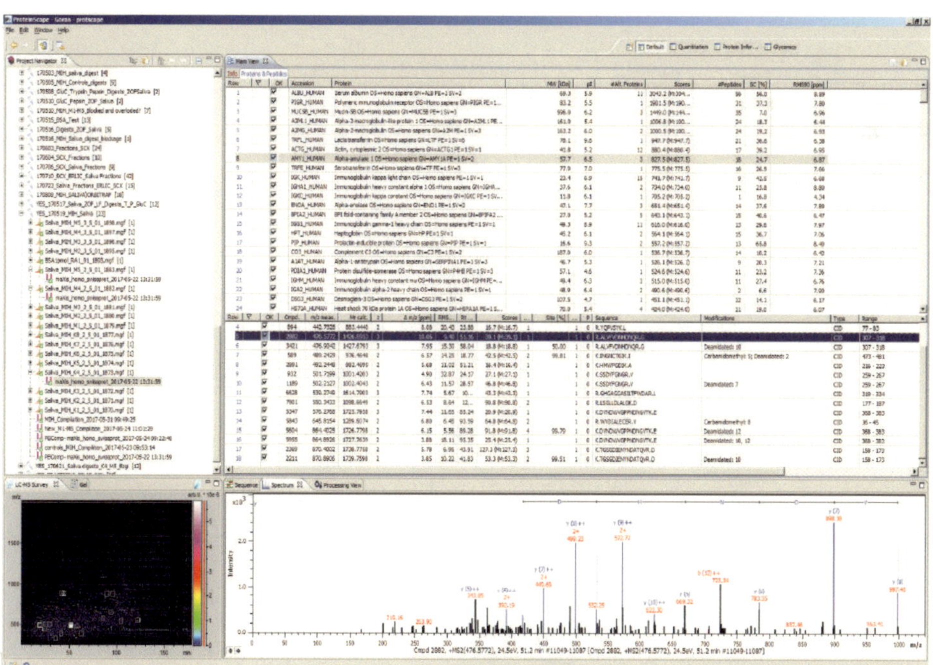

ProteinScape

Figure 6. Screenshots showing analysis of a salivary sample by applying two distinct software packages. Note that identified proteins have been listed based on their scores, which can be calculated using different algorithms.

Term	RT	Genes	Count	%	P-Value	FDR
Salivary secretion	RT		37	1.2	6.3E-9	8.4E-6
Glycolysis / Gluconeogenesis	RT		27	0.9	4.5E-6	6.0E-3
Carbon metabolism	RT		35	1.2	9.6E-5	1.3E-1
ABC transporters	RT		18	0.6	2.2E-4	2.9E-1
Glutamatergic synapse	RT		34	1.1	2.7E-4	3.6E-1
Biosynthesis of antibiotics	RT		54	1.8	3.3E-4	4.3E-1
Amoebiasis	RT		32	1.1	3.4E-4	4.5E-1
Oocyte meiosis	RT		32	1.1	5.8E-4	7.7E-1
Calcium signaling pathway	RT		45	1.5	1.5E-3	1.9E0
Platelet activation	RT		34	1.1	3.2E-3	4.2E0
Pathogenic Escherichia coli infection	RT		17	0.6	4.2E-3	5.4E0
Biosynthesis of amino acids	RT		22	0.7	4.4E-3	5.7E0
Regulation of actin cytoskeleton	RT		49	1.6	4.9E-3	6.4E0
Vascular smooth muscle contraction	RT		31	1.0	5.3E-3	6.9E0
Chemokine signaling pathway	RT		44	1.5	5.6E-3	7.2E0
Circadian entrainment	RT		26	0.9	5.9E-3	7.5E0
Endocytosis	RT		57	1.9	7.2E-3	9.2E0
Renin secretion	RT		19	0.6	8.8E-3	1.1E1
Pancreatic secretion	RT		25	0.8	8.9E-3	1.1E1
Pentose phosphate pathway	RT		11	0.4	1.1E-2	1.3E1
Arrhythmogenic right ventricular cardiomyopathy (ARVC)	RT		20	0.7	1.3E-2	1.6E1
GnRH signaling pathway	RT		24	0.8	1.3E-2	1.6E1
Tight junction	RT		33	1.1	1.3E-2	1.6E1
Oxytocin signaling pathway	RT		37	1.2	1.3E-2	1.6E1
Estrogen signaling pathway	RT		25	0.8	1.9E-2	2.3E1
Adrenergic signaling in cardiomyocytes	RT		34	1.1	1.9E-2	2.3E1
Dilated cardiomyopathy	RT		22	0.7	2.0E-2	2.3E1
Cholinergic synapse	RT		27	0.9	2.3E-2	2.7E1
Aldosterone synthesis and secretion	RT		21	0.7	2.6E-2	2.9E1
ECM-receptor interaction	RT		22	0.7	2.9E-2	3.2E1

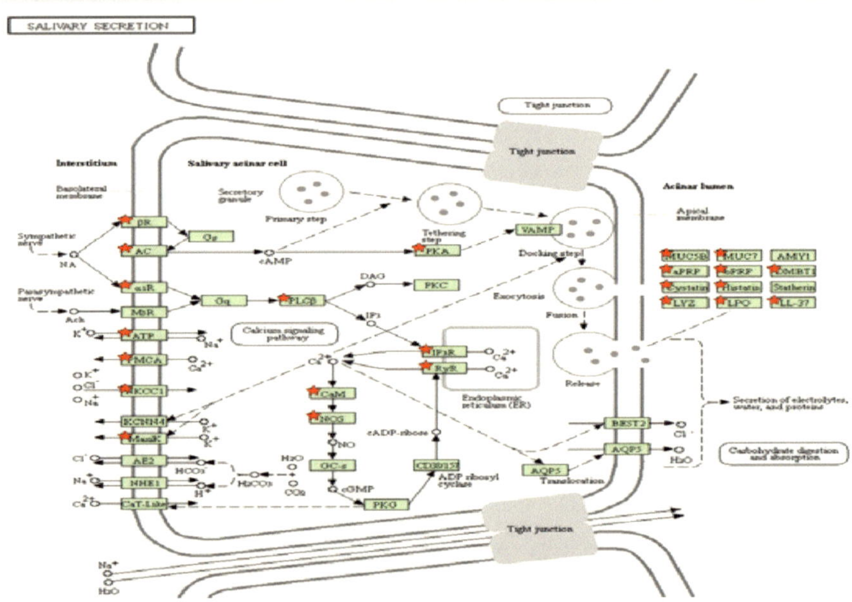

Figure 7. Pathway analysis of salivary proteins using DAVID® resulted in expected output and identification of *salivary secretion* as the pathway with the highest number of expressed proteins. Data courtesy of Zofia Świątczak (Master Thesis).

An exemplary result of the pathway analysis of a salivary sample using DAVID® is shown in **Figure 7**.

Finally, the analysis of all generated data and extracted information shall enable detection of putative biomarkers for diseases and therapy monitoring.

6. Application of salivary proteomics analysis for clinical research

As already mentioned, analysis of the salivary proteome can be applied to study a large area of conditions and diseases. The most intensively studied area of saliva as a diagnostic tool was its appliance for dental [21, 57, 64, 65], oral cancer [31, 66], diabetes [67, 68] or gastric cancer [58]. Furthermore, salivary proteomics was also applied for studying neurological and psychiatric disorders [69].

6.1. Application of salivary proteomics for diagnostics of oral diseases

The use of proteomics for diagnostics and treatment of oral diseases has been described in a number of publications. Jancsik et al. [70] describe the use of salivary proteomics to identify squamous oral cancer in diabetes patients. Authors have performed an additional sample homogenization, which is rarely described in other approaches to analyze saliva. Following analysis was performed by applying 2D gel separation of proteins and MS analysis using MALDI-TOF without the previous chromatographic separation and fractionation of proteins. It is known that inflammatory processes have a well-documented carcinogenetic role. Patients suffering from type-2 diabetes have also a higher risk of inflammatory diseases in the gastro-intestinal tract such as ulcerative colitis or Crohn's disease. These patients have also a higher risk of developing gastrointestinal cancer. It was shown that the incidence of developing benign tumors, leukoplakia, and malignancies was significantly increased in the group of patients with diabetes than in the healthy control group. The authors have shown a discovery of several putative biomarkers such as, e.g. Annexin A8-like, Annexin A8-like 1, Tyrosine kinase, AX969656, Protein kinase, Peroxiredoxin-2, and Annexin A2. Annexins are known to be overexpressed in colorectal cancer but also to have altered in tumorigenesis in several types of tumor. Furthermore, loss of Annexin A1 has been found to be an early event in esophageal squamous cell carcinoma. Obviously, these results show that diabetic patients have a higher risk of developing esophageal squamous cell carcinoma than the control healthy group and close monitoring shall be applied for early detection.

Delaleu et al. [71] have performed a particularly interesting and thorough investigation of the salivary proteome from patients suffering from Sjörgen's syndrome. Salivary proteome was analyzed using a 187-plex capture antibody-based assay, and the salivary proteomic biomarker profiles were generated from patients with primary Sjörgen's syndrome, patients with rheumatoid arthritis, and from asymptomatic controls. Authors were able to characterize putative biomarkers by detecting significant changes in 61 and 55 proteins, respectively, in samples of patients compared to that of donors without the diagnosis of Sjörgen's syndrome. Authors were able to detect, based on 4-plex and 6-plex biomarker signatures, markers including interleukin-4 (IL-4), IL-5, and clusterin. Accurate prediction of an individual's group membership was achieved for at least 94% of cases.

Winck et al. [72] analyzed the salivary proteome in order to decipher the immune response in oral cancer based on the salivary proteome and the extracellular vesicles isolated from saliva. The authors were able to identify significant differences in processes related to inflammatory and humoral immune responses, to peptidase inhibitor activity, iron coordination, and protease binding. Based on identifications achieved, the two classes of individuals (healthy versus patients with Oral Squamous Cell Carcinoma) were distinguished with 90% accuracy based solely on the proteomics data. The authors have used the label-free approach to quantify the identified proteins. Although both groups of peptides share the great majority of identified proteins, some identified proteins were present only in the healthy or only in the group diagnosed with cancer. Authors described that out of many differentially expressed proteins, only the protein peptidyl-prolyl cis-trans isomerase A (also known as cyclophilin-A) was statistically significant in the analysis of the mean survival time of patients, with reduced abundance of PPIA being a factor that may predict poor prognosis of OSCC patients.

6.2. Application of salivary proteomics for diagnostics of diabetes

Sedentary lifestyle paired with unhealthy food, environmental derogation, and stress situations have led to significant increase in diabetes patients worldwide. Early detection of biomarkers would enable more efficient therapy and possible delay of the diseases onset or even a prevention of the outbreak. Caseiro et al. [67] have described the use of proteomics to study Diabetes mellitus (DM) type-1. Authors have performed a quantitative proteomics analysis using the chemical proteomics approach and chemical labeling using iTRAQ. Here, sample from patients diagnosed with diabetes and from healthy subjects was pooled and processed prior to LC-MS/MS measurement and bioinformatics analysis of generated data. In addition to performing iTRAQ labeling and quantitation, authors have chosen for separating peptides by applying two-dimensional separation using high pH reversed phase chromatography. It is remarkable that authors also identified endogenous salivary peptides that are mostly ignored using MALDI-TOF and combined the results to identify more than 400 proteins. Authors used the data obtained to evaluate protein expression for patients with retinopathy, nephropathy, and no complications with the salivary proteome of healthy donors. Identification of the bactericidal/permeability increasing protein-like 1 (BPI) and pancreatic adenocarcinoma upregulated factor (PAUF) in the saliva of all diabetics clearly suggests that the activation of the immune system in type 1 DM is the most prominent process. One of the proteins, BPI, is an essential component of the innate immune system with bacteriostatic and bactericidal effects against gram-negative bacteria through lipopolysaccharides binding. The PAUF is an endogenous ligand of Toll-like receptor 2 (TLR2) and Toll-like receptor 4 (TLR4), and it is also involved in the inflammatory response, which seems to be more pronounced and more prominent in patients with retinopathy and nephropathy considering the high salivary levels of alpha-2-macroglobulin, defensin alpha 3 neutrophil-specific, leukocyte elastase inhibitor, matrix metalloproteinase-9, and neutrophil elastase.

As authors also performed analysis of the peptidome, interesting data were obtained that supported the hypothesis that Diabetes Mellitus (DM)-related proteins have higher susceptibility to proteolysis and evidenced an increased content of some specific protein fragments in saliva, which have been shown to be related with bacterial attachment and the accumulation of phosphopeptides. Especially, the accumulation of phosphopeptides seems to be involved in tooth protection against erosion and the level of their expression and phosphorylation might be a measure for dental damage that can be sustained in diabetes patients. The proteolytic fragments from bPRP1, bPRP2, and aPRP, in particular, might be considered for monitoring the disease pathogenesis with potential use for as early detection markers.

Rao et al. [73] applied multidimensional HPLC-MS/MS proteomics analysis for investigation of salivary proteins in patients with Diabetes Mellitus type-2. A Strong Cation Exchange separation of tryptic peptides from saliva of diabetic, prediabetic, and healthy subjects was performed prior to reversed phase separation and MS/MS detection. More than 400 proteins were identified and characterized and label-free quantitation was applied. As with other analysis, proteins involved with metabolic and inflammatory processes were detected in the saliva of subjects with diabetes. An important finding of the study was achieved in the prediabetic saliva: Salivary biomarkers of established Diabetes Mellitus were identified by proteomic profiling to be also differentially abundant in the saliva of patients with impaired glucose tolerance (IGT) alone and IGT + IFG (impaired fructose tolerance). These results were further confirmed by direct Western immunoblot and ELISA analyses.

The authors showed that the relative increase of some of these putative markers is associated with progression of prediabetes to the diabetic state. Therefore, systematic analysis of these putative biomarkers in prediabetic saliva, as well as their variability in individual samples, by immunoassays is of extreme importance for early acting and treatment of patients, which can prevent cardiovascular complications and mortality in diabetes patients.

An important aspect of patients suffering from DM type-2 is the severe retinopathy that can lead to blindness. Chee et al. [74] performed quantitative proteomics analysis of salivary proteins from patients diagnosed with DM type-2 without retinopathy, which served as controls and patients with DM type-2 and retinopathy. Quantitative proteomics analysis was performed by applying iTRAQ labeling and peptide separation before MS/MS detection was performed on a 50-cm nano column. Authors identified more than 300 proteins but have selected only the fully labeled pairs for quantitative analysis, a total of 119 proteins. Authors identified that increased proteins were predicted to be defense proteins and metabolic proteins suggesting that the expression of salivary defense and metabolic proteins is related to diabetic retinopathy. These results confirmed the report by Fernandez-Real et al. [75] that defense response proteins were elevated in type-2 diabetic patients and this gradually led to surging of metabolic proteins.

6.3. Application of salivary proteomics for psychiatric and neurological diseases

Fields of neurology and psychiatry urgently need new biomarkers for objective and earlier diagnoses of conditions attributed to the central nervous system (CNS). Proteomics and other "omics" technologies are being increasingly applied for these discoveries. Henskens et al. [76] performed analysis of salivary proteins already in 1996 for patients treated with different medications for epilepsy. This work was not performed by using nowadays technology, however, several salivary proteins in saliva from epileptic patients, who were medicated with different antiepileptic drugs (namely phenytoin, valproate, and carbamazepine), were found to be increased and were compared with protein levels in the saliva of healthy control subjects. It was also found that, for all patient groups, the specific amylase activity was increased up to twofold. On the other side, absolute and relative concentrations of cystatin S were diminished in all samples, but particularly strong in patients using either valproate or phenytoin. These data suggest that use of antiepileptic drugs over long periods may cause a decrease of salivary proteins such as sIgA and cystatins, which are involved in the protection of the oral cavity against microbial infections and, therefore, these patients suffer more complications related to gingiva and oral cavity in general.

Ngounou Wetie et al. [77] have investigated the use of salivary proteins as possible markers for early onset of Autism Spectrum Disorders (ASDs). Authors have identified increased levels of apolipoproteins apoA1 and apoA4 and of serum paraoxonase/arylesterase 1 (PON1) in ASD sera compared to healthy controls in blood serum and have tested the hypothesis that levels of these peptides might also be elevated in saliva. Authors found statistically significant differences in expression of a number of salivary proteins such as elevated prolactin-inducible protein, lactotransferrin, Ig kappa chain C region, Ig gamma-1 chain C region, Ig lambda-2 chain C regions, neutrophil elastase, polymeric immunoglobulin receptor and deleted in malignant brain tumors 1. Identifications made support the hypothesis that immune system disturbances may be present in individuals with ASDs.

Castagnola et al. [78, 79] have applied a proteomics approach for studying the naturally occurring peptidome of human saliva in children diagnosed with ASDs. The study revealed that naturally occurring peptides in the saliva of children with ASD can bear multiple phosphorylations. The phosphorylation level of four specific salivary phosphopeptides, identified in this study, statherin, histatin 1, and acidic proline-rich proteins for both entire and truncated isoforms, was found to be significantly lower in autistic patients, with hypophosphorylation of at least one peptide observed in 18 ASD subjects (66%). Authors suggest that different phosphorylation and hypophosphorylation of salivary peptides suggest potential asynchronies in the phosphorylation of other secretory proteins. These proteins could be relevant in the development of central nervous system during embryonic development or in early infancy. Furthermore, obtained results suggest that naturally occurring salivary phosphopeptides might help to detect and discriminate a subgroup of ASD patients.

6.4. Application of salivary proteomics for dentistry

Saliva has a continuous and intensive contact and interaction with human teeth and plays an important role in cleaning the tooth surface and antimicrobial defense. Salivary proteomics and its role in dentistry have been studied in a number of experiments. Some of these have addressed the role of salivary proteins in edentulous patients diagnosed with DM. Byrd et al. and Border et al. [80, 81] have addressed the problem of edentulous patients with Denture stomatitis (DS) and DM type-2.

Denture stomatitis refers to an inflammatory condition of the mucosal tissue underneath the denture, which could lead to severe health problems. Clinical classification of DS distinguishes three types: type 1 (DS I), type 2 (DS II), and type 3 (DS III), referring to clinically localized mild, localized moderate, and generalized tissue inflammation [80]. Authors have performed a quantitative proteomics analysis based on label-free quantitation and using two different MS platforms—an Orbitrap instrument and a Time-of-flight instrument. Interestingly, proteins were detected as differentially expressed between the two LC/MS systems. Protein expression was also different depending on the severity of DS. Authors have observed different levels of protein expression between different stages of DS and between the number of identified and quantified proteins for different disease stages and have identified serum proteins in the saliva of patients with DS III, e.g. ceruloplasmin, hemoglobins, serotransferrin, and albumin, which suggest that DS III patients experience higher level of inflammation and protein leakage from blood into saliva.

An interesting approach has been undertaken by Kaczor-Urbanowicz et al. [82] to study tooth absorption during an inflammatory process caused by orthodontic tooth movement. The orthodontically induced inflammatory root resorption (OIIRR) occurs as a consequence (the most prevalent and unavoidable) of orthodontic tooth movement. Authors have applied 2D-gel separation for salivary proteins upon depletion of abundant proteins (amylase, serum albumin, and IgG), and separated the tryptic peptides using HPLC followed by MS/MS detection. Identified proteins were quantified using the label-free approach. Authors were able to identify more than 700 proteins, which were revealed by quantitative MS of which different numbers were identified for different groups of patients. The strength of this study lays with the depth of the analyzed proteome and the significance of the results. Authors performed the bioinformatic analysis for proteins, which were found to be more than threefold increased. Different patient groups revealed different results although they all have been diagnosed with the tooth resorption. The moderate-to-severe root resorption young group revealed 38 functional clusters associated with acute and dynamic processes and in the moderate-to-severe root resorption adult group, other 16 functional clusters were found and those were related to less dynamic and slower processes. For the young group, these processes included the regulation of acute inflammatory response, defense response, response to stress, response to wounding or healing as opposed to apoptosis, glycoproteins expression, cell adhesion, signal peptides, etc. in the adult group with moderate-to-severe processes. Finally, a number of new putative biomarkers were identified, and these might be used to produce a clinical test that would serve along with radiography to perform a fast and more reliable diagnosis.

7. Conclusion

In summary, salivary proteomics is an upcoming approach for both basic and clinical research with a significant potential for use in fast diagnostic approaches. Not only the analysis of salivary proteins but also the analysis of endogenous peptides in saliva and their posttranslational modifications shall be addressed and targeted. Although a number of studies have been published and more are to come, more research is required to validate the discovered putative biomarkers so far.

Current proteomics approach for the analysis of oral fluid is not yet suited for daily routine in clinical diagnostics. However, it can help discovering biomarkers for which immunological tests such as ELISA can be developed.

Furthermore, it is essential to develop and curate a comprehensive database for the salivary proteome and establish standard conditions for sample collection and processing until the MS analysis.

The space was scarce in this chapter to address more of the clinical approach of salivary proteomics, but the researcher is encouraged to stay focused and follow the further development.

Current development shows that, without any doubt, this process will continue and will yield more biomarker candidates in the future.

Author details

Goran Mitulović

Address all correspondence to: goran.mitulovic@meduniwien.ac.at

Medical University of Vienna, Clinical Department of Laboratory Medicine, Vienna, Austria

References

[1] Bianchi L, Gagliardi A, Landi C, Focarelli R, De Leo V, Luddi A, et al. Protein pathways working in human follicular fluid: The future for tailored IVF? Expert Reviews in Molecular Medicine. 2016;**18**:e9

[2] Huang G, Zhou C, Wei C-J, Zhao S, Sun F, Zhou H, et al. Evaluation of in vitro fertilization outcomes using interleukin-8 in culture medium of human preimplantation embryos. Fertility and Sterility. 2017;**107**(3):649-656

[3] Corbo C, Cevenini A, Salvatore F. Biomarker discovery by proteomics-based approaches for early detection and personalized medicine in colorectal cancer. Proteomics—Clinical Applications. 2017;**11**(5-6):n/a

[4] Nkuipou-Kenfack E, Zürbig P, Mischak H. The long path towards implementation of clinical proteomics: Exemplified based on CKD273. Proteomics—Clinical Applications. 2017;**11**(5-6):n/a

[5] Cifani P, Kentsis A. Towards comprehensive and quantitative proteomics for diagnosis and therapy of human disease. Proteomics. 2017;**17**(1-2):160079

[6] Kasprzyk J, Stępień E, Piekoszewski W. Application of nano-LC-MALDI-TOF/TOF-MS for proteomic analysis of microvesicles. Clinical Biochemistry. 2017;**50**(4-5):241-243

[7] Vaudel M, Sickmann A, Martens L. Introduction to opportunities and pitfalls in functional mass spectrometry based proteomics. Biochimica et Biophysica Acta (BBA)—Proteins and Proteomics. 2014;**1844**(1, Part A):12-20

[8] Pehar M. Changes in protein expression and lysine acetylation induced by decreased glutathione levels in astrocytes. Molecular & Cellular Proteomics. 2016;**15**:493-505

[9] Gu H. Quantitative profiling of post-translational modifications by immunoaffinity enrichment and LC-MS/MS in cancer serum without Immunodepletion. Molecular & Cellular Proteomics. 2016;**15**:692-702

[10] Broncel M. Global profiling of Huntingtin-associated protein E (HYPE)-mediated AMPylation through a chemical proteomic approach. Molecular & Cellular Proteomics. 2016;**15**:715-725

[11] Hutter G, Sailer M, Azad TD, von Bueren AO, Nollau P, Frank S, et al. Reverse phase protein arrays enable glioblastoma molecular subtyping. Journal of Neuro-Oncology. 2017;**131**(3):437-448

[12] Cifani P, Kentsis A. Towards comprehensive and quantitative proteomics for diagnosis and therapy of human disease. Proteomics. 2017;**17**(1-2):160079

[13] Oluwadara O, Chiappelli F. Biomarkers for early detection of high risk cancers: From gliomas to nasopharyngeal carcinoma. Bioinformation. 2009;**3**(8):332-339

[14] Debald M, Wolfgarten M, Walgenbach-Brunagel G, Kuhn W, Braun M. Non-invasive proteomics-thinking about personalized breast cancer screening and treatment. The EPMA Journal. 2010;**1**(3):413-420

[15] Wistuba II, Gelovani JG, Jacoby JJ, Davis SE, Herbst RS. Methodological and practical challenges for personalized cancer therapies. Nature Reviews. Clinical Oncology. 2011;**8**

[16] Baum BJ, Yates JR 3rd, Srivastava S, Wong DT, Melvin JE. Scientific frontiers: Emerging technologies for salivary diagnostics. Advances in Dental Research. 2011;**23**(4):360-368

[17] Haynes H, Camelo-Piragua S, Kurian K. Prognostic and predictive biomarkers in adult and pediatric gliomas: Toward personalized treatment. Frontiers in Oncology. 2014;**4**(47)

[18] Li BT, Lou E, Hsu M, HA Y, Naidoo J, Zauderer MG, et al. Serum biomarkers associated with clinical outcomes fail to predict brain metastases in patients with stage IV non-small cell lung cancers. PLoS One. 2016;**11**(1):e0146063

[19] Luhtala N, Aslanian A, Yates JR 3rd, Hunter T. Secreted glioblastoma nanovesicles contain intracellular signaling proteins and active Ras incorporated in a farnesylation-dependent manner. The Journal of Biological Chemistry. 2017;**292**(2):611-628

[20] Tang Z, Louie RF, Kost G, Kost N. Principles and Practice of Point-of-Care Testing. 2002. Lippincott Williams & Wilkins

[21] Wong DT. Salivary diagnostics powered by nanotechnologies, proteomics and genomics. Journal of the American Dental Association (1939). 2006;**137**(3):313-321

[22] Zhang L, Henson BS, Camargo PM, Wong DT. The clinical value of salivary biomarkers for periodontal disease. Periodontology 2000. 2009;**51**:25-37

[23] Chin CD, Chin SY, Laksanasopin T, Sia SK, Issadore D, Westervelt RM. Point-of-Care Diagnostics on a Chip. 2013. 3 p

[24] Aro K, Wei F, Wong DT, Tu M. saliva liquid biopsy for point-of-care applications. Frontiers in Public Health. 2017;**5**

[25] Pusch W, Flocco MT, Leung SM, Thiele H, Kostrzewa M. Mass spectrometry-based clinical proteomics. Pharmacogenomics. 2003;**4**(4):463-476

[26] Huang CM. Comparative proteomic analysis of human whole saliva. Archives of Oral Biology. 2004;**49**(12):951-962

[27] Xie H, Rhodus NL, Griffin RJ, Carlis JV, Griffin TJ. A catalogue of human saliva proteins identified by free flow electrophoresis-based peptide separation and tandem mass spectrometry. Molecular & Cellular Proteomics. 2005;**4**(11):1826-1830

[28] Streckfus C, Bigler L. The use of soluble, salivary c-erbB-2 for the detection and postoperative follow-up of breast cancer in women: The results of a five-year translational research study. Advances in Dental Research. 2005;**18**(1):17-24

[29] Al Kawas S, Rahim ZH, Ferguson DB. Potential uses of human salivary protein and peptide analysis in the diagnosis of disease. Archives of Oral Biology. 2012;**57**(1):1-9

[30] Yoshizawa JM, Schafer CA, Schafer JJ, Farrell JJ, Paster BJ, Wong DT. Salivary biomarkers: Toward future clinical and diagnostic utilities. Clinical Microbiology Reviews. 2013;**26**

[31] Krishna Prasad RB, Sharma A, Babu HM. An insight into salivary markers in oral cancer. Dental Research Journal. 2013;**10**(3):287-295

[32] Kaczor-Urbanowicz KE, Martin Carreras-Presas C, Aro K, Tu M, Garcia-Godoy F, Wong DT. Saliva diagnostics—Current views and directions. Experimental Biology and Medicine. 2017;**242**(5):459-472

[33] Sun Y, Liu S, Qiao Z, Shang Z, Xia Z, Niu X, et al. Systematic comparison of exosomal proteomes from human saliva and serum for the detection of lung cancer. Analytica Chimica Acta. 2017;**982**:84-95

[34] Carro E, Bartolome F, Bermejo-Pareja F, Villarejo-Galende A, Molina JA, Ortiz P, et al. Early diagnosis of mild cognitive impairment and Alzheimer's disease based on salivary lactoferrin. Alzheimer's & Dementia (Amsterdam, Netherlands). 2017;**8**:131-138

[35] Kochurova EV, Nikolenko VN. Estimation of expression of oral fluid biomarkers in the diagnosis of Pretumor diseases of oral mucosa. Bulletin of Experimental Biology and Medicine. 2017;**163**(1):87-91

[36] Aqrawi LA, Galtung HK, Vestad B, Ovstebo R, Thiede B, Rusthen S, et al. Identification of potential saliva and tear biomarkers in primary Sjogren's syndrome, utilising the extraction of extracellular vesicles and proteomics analysis. Arthritis Research & Therapy. 2017;**19**(1):14

[37] Slowey PD. Salivary diagnostics using purified nucleic acids. Methods in Molecular Biology. 2017;**1537**:3-15

[38] Kaczor-Urbanowicz KE, Martin Carreras-Presas C, Aro K, Tu M, Garcia-Godoy F, Wong DT. Saliva diagnostics—Current views and directions. Experimental Biology and Medicine (Maywood, NJ). 2017;**242**(5):459-472

[39] Kaczor-Urbanowicz KE, Martin Carreras-Presas C, Kaczor T, Tu M, Wei F, Garcia-Godoy F, et al. Emerging technologies for salivaomics in cancer detection. Journal of Cellular and Molecular Medicine. 2017;**21**(4):640-647

[40] Coucke LD, De Smet L, Verstraete AG. Influence of sampling procedure on codeine concentrations in oral fluid. Journal of Analytical Toxicology. 2016;**40**(2):148-152

[41] Deeley K, Noel J, Vieira AR. Comparative study of five commercially available saliva collection kits for DNA extraction. Clinical Laboratory. 2016;**62**(9):1809-1813

[42] Rapp-Santos KJ, Altamura LA, Norris SL, Lugo-Roman LA, Rico PJ, Hofer CC. Comparison of saliva collection methods for the determination of salivary cortisol levels in rhesus macaques (*Macaca mulatta*), Cynomolgus macaques (*Macaca fascicularis*), and African green monkeys (*Chlorocebus aethiops*). Journal of the American Association for Laboratory Animal Science : JAALAS. 2017

[43] Roth R, Baxter J, Vehik K, Hopkins D, Killian M, Gesualdo P, et al. The feasibility of salivary sample collection in an international pediatric cohort: The the TEDDY study. Developmental Psychobiology. 2017;**59**(5):658-667

[44] Chetwynd AJ, Dunn WB, Rodriguez-Blanco G. Collection and preparation of clinical samples for metabolomics. Advances in Experimental Medicine and Biology. 2017;**965**:19-44

[45] Cohier C, Megarbane B, Roussel O. Illicit drugs in oral fluid: Evaluation of two collection devices. Journal of Analytical Toxicology. 2017;**41**(1):71-76

[46] Groschl M, Kohler H, Topf HG, Rupprecht T, Rauh M. Evaluation of saliva collection devices for the analysis of steroids, peptides and therapeutic drugs. Journal of Pharmaceutical and Biomedical Analysis. 2008;**47**(3):478-486

[47] Lundy FT, Lamey PJ. The recovery of proteolytic activity using the Salivette system. European Journal of Clinical Chemistry and Clinical Biochemistry: Journal of the Forum of European Clinical Chemistry Societies. 1995;**33**(7):443-444

[48] Lamey PJ, Nolan A. The recovery of human saliva using the Salivette system. European Journal of Clinical Chemistry and Clinical Biochemistry: Journal of the Forum of European Clinical Chemistry Societies. 1994;**32**(9):727-728

[49] Chiang SH, Thomas GA, Liao W, Grogan T, Buck RL, Fuentes L, et al. RNAPro*SAL: A device for rapid and standardized collection of saliva RNA and proteins. BioTechniques. 2015;**58**(2):69-76

[50] Golatowski C, Gesell Salazar M, Dhople VM, Hammer E, Kocher T, Jehmlich N, et al. Comparative evaluation of saliva collection methods for proteome analysis. Clinica Chimica Acta. 2013;**419**:42-46

[51] Jambunathan K, Galande AK. Sample collection in clinical proteomics—Proteolytic activity profile of serum and plasma. Proteomics—Clinical Applications. 2014:n/a

[52] Torregrossa AM, Nikonova L, Bales MB, Leal MV, Smith JC, Contreras RJ, et al. Induction of salivary proteins modifies measures of both orosensory and postingestive feedback during exposure to a tannic acid diet. PLoS One. 2014;**9**(8)

[53] Wessel D, Flügge UI. A method for the quantitative recovery of protein in dilute solution in the presence of detergents and lipids. Analytical Biochemistry. 1984;**138**(1):141-143

[54] Fichtenbaum A, Schmid R, Mitulović G. Direct injection of HILIC fractions on the reversed phase trap column improves protein identification rates for salivary proteins. Electrophoresis. 2016;**37**(22):2922-2929

[55] Meyer JG, Kim S, Maltby D, Ghassemian M, Bandeira N, Komives EA. Expanding proteome coverage with orthogonal-specificity alpha-lytic proteases. Molecular & Cellular Proteomics. 2014

[56] Brownridge P, Beynon RJ. The importance of the digest: Proteolysis and absolute quantification in proteomics. Methods. 2011;**54**(4):351-360

[57] Deutsch O, Fleissig Y, Zaks B, Krief G, Aframian DJ, Palmon A. An approach to remove alpha amylase for proteomic analysis of low abundance biomarkers in human saliva. Electrophoresis. 2008;**29**(20):4150-4157

[58] Xiao H, Zhang Y, Kim Y, Kim S, Kim JJ, Kim KM, et al. Differential proteomic analysis of human saliva using tandem mass tags quantification for gastric cancer detection. Scientific Reports. 2016;**6**:22165

[59] Tarasova IA, Lobas AA, Černigoj U, Solovyeva EM, Mahlberg B, Ivanov MV, et al. Depletion of human serum albumin in embryo culture media for in vitro fertilization using monolithic columns with immobilized antibodies. Electrophoresis. 2016;**37**(17-18): 2322-2327

[60] Mitulović G, Smoluch M, Chervet J-P, Steinmacher I, Kungl A, Mechtler K. An improved method for tracking and reducing the void volume in nano HPLC–MS with micro trapping columns. Analytical and Bioanalytical Chemistry. 2003;**376**(7):946-951

[61] Alpert AJ. Electrostatic repulsion hydrophilic interaction chromatography for isocratic separation of charged solutes and selective isolation of phosphopeptides. Analytical Chemistry. 2007;**80**(1):62-76

[62] Hao P, Qian J, Dutta B, Cheow ESH, Sim KH, Meng W, et al. Enhanced separation and characterization of deamidated peptides with RP-ERLIC-based multidimensional chromatography coupled with tandem mass spectrometry. Journal of Proteome Research. 2012;**11**(3):1804-1811

[63] Mitulovic G, Stingl C, Smoluch M, Swart R, Chervet JP, Steinmacher I, et al. Automated, on-line two-dimensional nano liquid chromatography tandem mass spectrometry for rapid analysis of complex protein digests. Proteomics. 2004;**4**(9):2545-2557

[64] Moffa EB, Machado MA, Mussi MC, Xiao Y, Garrido SS, Giampaolo ET, et al. Vitro identification of Histatin 5 salivary complexes. PLoS One. 2015;**10**(11):e0142517

[65] Fleissig Y, Deutsch O, Reichenberg E, Redlich M, Zaks B, Palmon A, et al. Different proteomic protein patterns in saliva of Sjogren's syndrome patients. Oral Diseases. 2009;**15**(1):61-68

[66] Wu C-C, Chu H-W, Hsu C-W, Chang K-P, Liu H-P. Saliva proteome profiling reveals potential salivary biomarkers for detection of oral cavity squamous cell carcinoma. Proteomics. 2015;**15**(19):3394-3404

[67] Caseiro A, Ferreira R, Padrão A, Quintaneiro C, Pereira A, Marinheiro R, et al. Salivary proteome and peptidome profiling in type 1 diabetes mellitus using a quantitative approach. Journal of Proteome Research. 2013;**12**(4):1700-1709

[68] Bencharit S, Baxter SS, Carlson J, Byrd WC, Mayo MV, Border MB, et al. Salivary proteins associated with hyperglycemia in diabetes: A proteomic analysis. Molecular bioSystems. 2013;**9**(11):2785-2797

[69] Wormwood KL, Aslebagh R, Channaveerappa D, Dupree EJ, Borland MM, Ryan JP, et al. Salivary proteomics and biomarkers in neurology and psychiatry. Proteomics—Clinical Applications. 2015;**9**(9-10):899-906

[70] Jancsik VA, Gelencser G, Maasz G, Schmidt J, Molnar GA, Wittmann I, et al. Salivary proteomic analysis of diabetic patients for possible oral squamous cell carcinoma biomarkers. Pathology Oncology Research: POR. 2014;**20**(3):591-595

[71] Delaleu N, Mydel P, Kwee I, Brun JG, Jonsson MV, Jonsson R. High fidelity between saliva proteomics and the biologic state of salivary glands defines biomarker signatures for primary Sjogren's syndrome. Arthritis & rheumatology (Hoboken, NJ). 2015;**67**(4):1084-1095

[72] Winck FV, Prado Ribeiro AC, Ramos Domingues R, Ling LY, Riano-Pachon DM, Rivera C, et al. Insights into immune responses in oral cancer through proteomic analysis of saliva and salivary extracellular vesicles. Scientific Reports. 2015;**5**:16305

[73] Rao PV, Reddy AP, Lu X, Dasari S, Krishnaprasad A, Biggs E, et al. Proteomic identification of salivary biomarkers of Type-2 diabetes. Journal of Proteome Research. 2009;**8**(1):239-245

[74] Chee CS, Chang KM, Loke MF, Angela Loo VP, Subrayan V. Association of potential salivary biomarkers with diabetic retinopathy and its severity in type-2 diabetes mellitus: A proteomic analysis by mass spectrometry. PeerJ. 2016;**4**:e2022

[75] Fernandez-Real JM, Pickup JC. Innate immunity, insulin resistance and type 2 diabetes. Trends in Endocrinology and Metabolism: TEM. 2008;**19**(1):10-16

[76] Henskens YMC, Strooker H, van den Keijbus PAM, Veerman ECI, Nieuw Amerongen AV. Salivary protein composition in epileptic patients on different medications. Journal of Oral Pathology & Medicine. 1996;**25**(7):360-366

[77] Ngounou Wetie AG, Wormwood KL, Russell S, Ryan JP, Darie CC, Woods AGA. Pilot proteomic analysis of salivary biomarkers in autism spectrum disorder. Autism Research: Official Journal of the International Society for Autism Research. 2015;**8**(3):338-350

[78] Castagnola M, Scarano E, Passali GC, Messana I, Cabras T, Iavarone F, et al. Salivary biomarkers and proteomics: Future diagnostic and clinical utilities. Acta Otorhinolaryngologica Italica: Organo Ufficiale della Societa Italiana di Otorinolaringologia e Chirurgia Cervico-facciale. 2017;**37**(2):94-101

[79] Castagnola M, Messana I, Inzitari R, Fanali C, Cabras T, Morelli A, et al. Hypo-phosphorylation of salivary peptidome as a clue to the molecular pathogenesis of autism Spectrum disorders. Journal of Proteome Research. 2008;**7**(12):5327-5332

[80] Byrd WC, Schwartz-Baxter S, Carlson J, Barros S, Offenbacher S, Bencharit S. Role of salivary and candidal proteins in denture stomatitis: An exploratory proteomic analysis. Molecular bioSystems. 2014;**10**(9):2299-2304

[81] Border MB, Schwartz S, Carlson J, Dibble CF, Kohltfarber H, Offenbacher S, et al. Exploring salivary proteomes in edentulous patients with type 2 diabetes. Molecular bioSystems. 2012;**8**(4):1304-1310

[82] Kaczor-Urbanowicz KE, Deutsch O, Zaks B, Krief G, Chaushu S, Palmon A. Identification of salivary protein biomarkers for orthodontically induced inflammatory root resorption. Proteomics—Clinical Applications. 2017;**11**(9-10):1600119

Chapter 6

Approach to Diagnosis of Salivary Gland Disease from Nuclear Medicine Images

Michihiro Nakayama, Atsutaka Okizaki,
Kaori Nakajima and Koji Takahashi

Additional information is available at the end of the chapter

http://dx.doi.org/10.5772/intechopen.70622

Abstract

Nuclear medicine images can help in the diagnosis and assessment of some salivary disorders. 99mTcO4−, gallium-67-citrate scintigraphy will be an indication of the function of salivary gland together and it will be used for the diffuse diseases such as sialadenitis, Sjögren's syndrome, sarcoidosis, glossopharyngeal paralysis, and irradiation. It is also effective for distinguishing benign tumor legion with Warthin's tumor and others. Moreover, fluorodeoxyglucose positron emission tomography (FDG-PET) is an indispensable modality for determining the localization, focal lesions, and staging of many malignant tumors, the fluorodeoxyglucose (FDG) accumulation is visually and semi-quantitatively assessed using the standardized uptake value (SUV), which is the ratio of uptake to the injected dose per unit body weight. Also for radioactive iodine therapy, attention should be paid to adverse reactions. It is important to note that acute/chronic salivary gland disorders are associated with radioiodine therapy for the treatment of postoperative thyroid cancer. Coordination among healthcare providers including nurses, radiological technologists, and doctors of all departments involved in treatment is important for achieving effective outcomes.

Keywords: scintigraphy, 99mTcO4−, SPECT, FDG-PET, salivary gland disorders

1. Introduction

Radionuclide imaging, commonly used for the diagnosis of salivary gland diseases, consists of salivary scintigraphy using 99mTcO4−, gallium-67-citrate (67Ga) scintigraphy in inflammation, and fluorodeoxyglucose positron emission tomography (FDG-PET). It is important to note that acute/chronic salivary gland disorders are associated with radioiodine therapy for the treatment of postoperative thyroid cancer.

2. Salivary gland scintigraphy

2.1. Mechanism of uptake

Salivary glands secrete saliva. The parotid, submandibular, and sublingual glands are called the "major salivary glands." Salivary epithelial cells have a sodium/iodide symporter (NIS), which takes up univalent anions such as Cl– and I– and concentrates them (**Figure 1**). The concentrated anion is secreted into saliva. Administered 99mTcO4– (**Figure 2**) is taken up by the salivary glands through NIS, similar to Cl–. Thus, intravenously administered 99mTcO4– accumulates mainly in the parotid and submandibular glands and is excreted into saliva [1]. After the accumulation of the radionuclide, loading of citric acid, such as lemon juice, stimulates the secretion of saliva, which indicates salivary gland function. Salivary gland scintigraphy is useful for differentiating salivary gland tumors because Warthin's tumors and oncocytomas, which are benign, retain 99mTcO4–.

2.2. Testing procedure

Because salivary gland function is affected by food intake, 1 hour of fasting is needed before testing.

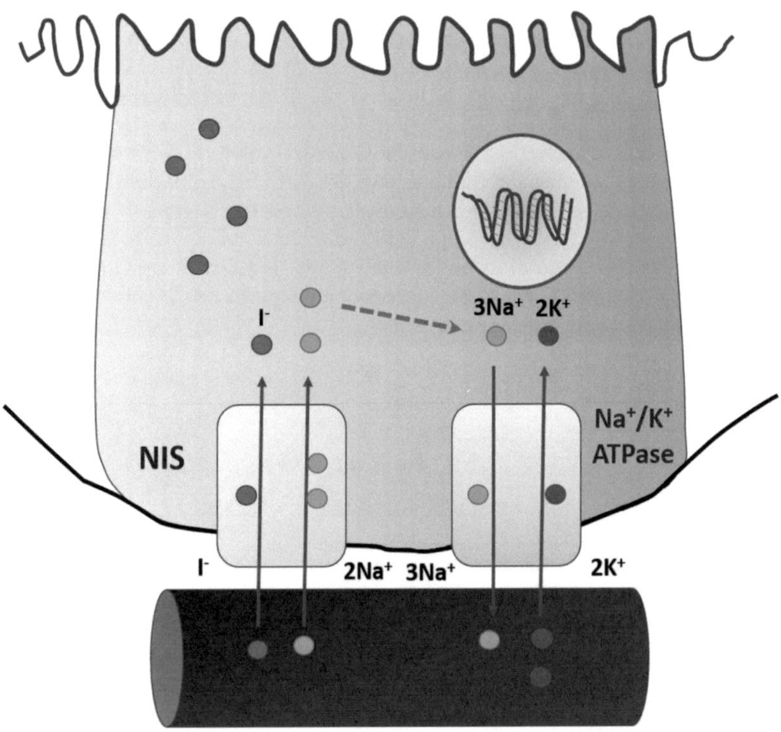

Figure 1. Iodide uptake mechanism of sodium/iodide symporter. Sodium/iodide symporter transports two sodium ions and one iodide ion into the cytoplasm together.

http://dx.doi.org/10.5772/intechopen.70622

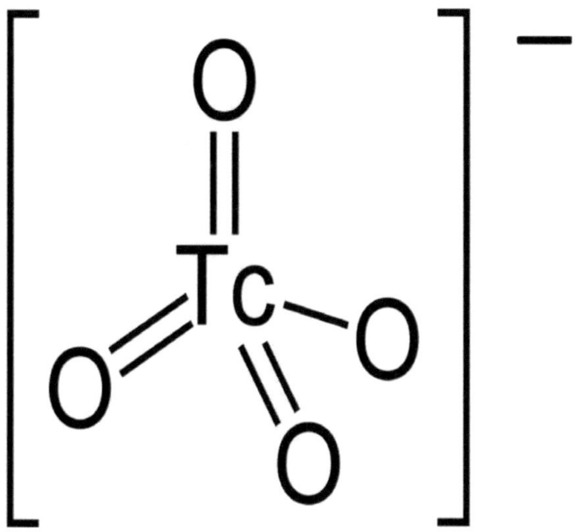

Figure 2. Structural formula of 99mTcO4–. 99mTcO4– is incorporated into the salivary glands through NIS, similar to Cl–.

For the kinetic analysis of salivary gland function, 185–370 MBq (5–10 mCi) of 99mTcO4– is intravenously administered. A dynamic scan (anteroposterior view) is performed at 5-minute intervals for 30 minutes. The thyroid gland should be included in the area. Citric acid (e.g., lemon juice) is instilled into the oral cavity 20 minutes after the intravenous injection to stimulate the secretion of saliva. The regions of interest are set at the bilateral parotid and submandibular glands, and at background regions to generate time-activity curves (TAC). The TAC is used to determine the function of individual salivary gland. For the diagnosis of tumors and morphology of salivary glands, the intravenously administered dose is 370–740 MBq, and the anteroposterior and lateral images are obtained 10–15 minutes after intravenous administration (**Figure 3**). When the assessment of the tumor is difficult due to the physiologic uptake in the normal salivary glands, washout by stimulating the secretion of saliva is useful.

2.3. Imaging evaluation

2.3.1. Normal images

Salivary gland scintigraphy provides information about the morphology and function of the salivary glands and the procedure is easier than that of sialography.

2.3.2. Dynamic scans and TAC

The uptake in the bilateral parotid and submandibular glands begins less than 1 minute after intravenous administration of the radionuclide and increases over time. The uptake in the parotid glands is equal to or greater than that in the submandibular glands. The sublingual glands are not visible, though the reason is unknown. After the stimulation of saliva secretion, the uptake rapidly declines in all four glands and subsequently rises again. The percentage

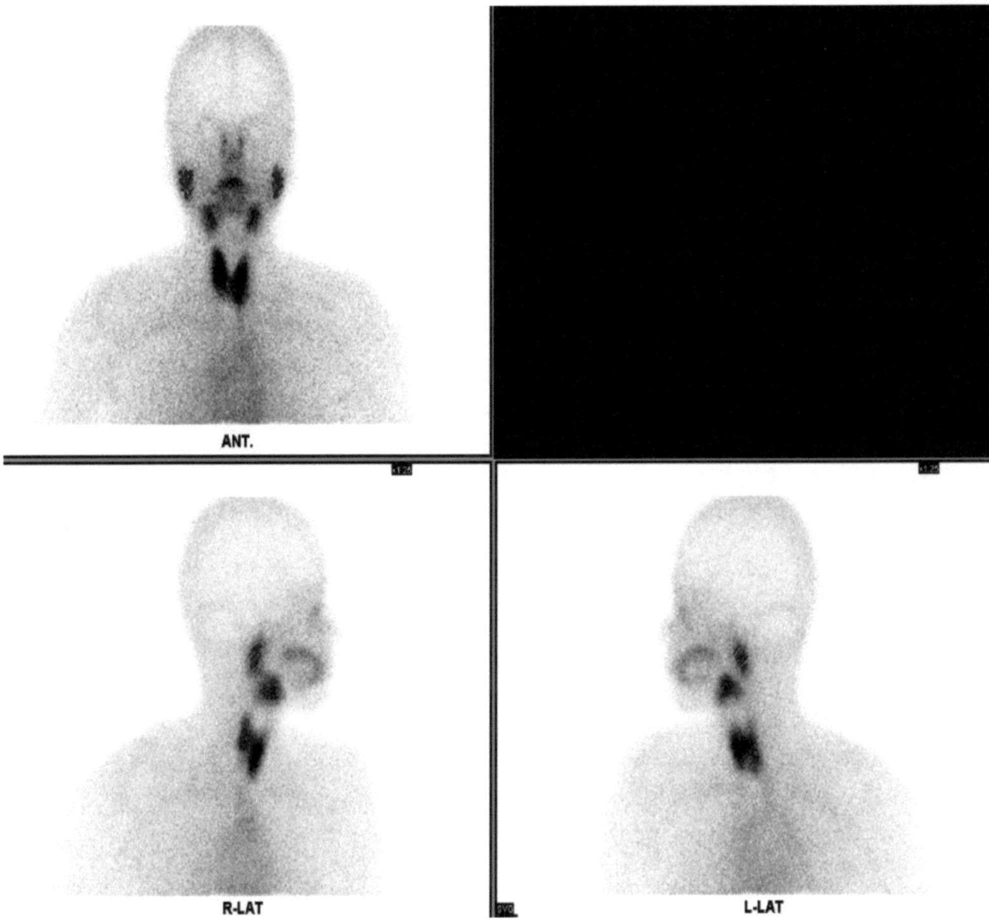

Figure 3. Static images in normal case. The radionuclide uptake of the parotid and submandibular glands is equal to or lower than that of the normal thyroid gland.

of washout is calculated using the counts at the maximum uptake and those at the minimum uptake seen after the stimulation of saliva secretion in each gland. The washout (%) is 50% or higher in the normal salivary gland (**Figure 4**).

2.3.3. Static images

The radionuclide uptake of the parotid and submandibular glands are equal to or lower than that of the normal thyroid gland, and mild uptake appears in the nasal and oral cavities. On the lateral view, the parotid gland is clearly shown, but the submandibular gland overlaps with the contralateral submandibular gland.

2.4. Diagnosis of salivary gland tumors

Warthin's tumors and oncocytomas are derived from the epithelial cells of excretory ducts and do not communicate via excretory ducts (**Figure 5**). Thus, 99mTcO4– is taken up by the

http://dx.doi.org/10.5772/intechopen.70622

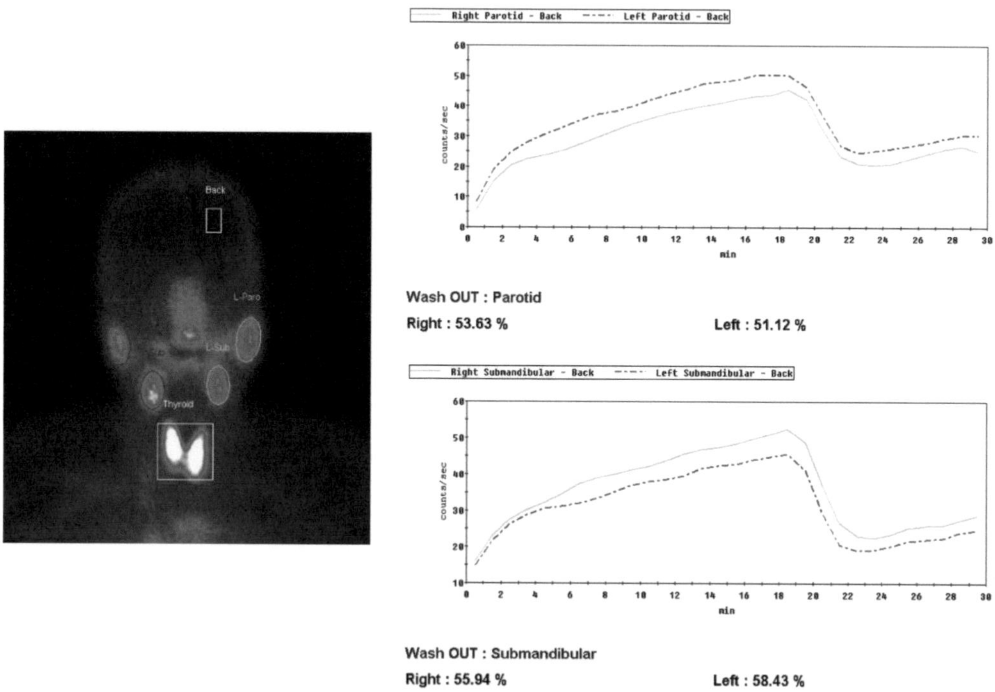

Figure 4. TAC of the normal salivary gland. After intravenous administration of the radionuclide, uptake in the parotid and submandibular glands increases over time. At 20 minutes after administration, saliva secretion is stimulated. Counts in the salivary glands rapidly decline and then gradually increase again.

solid component of these tumors and is not eliminated after the stimulation of saliva secretion. However, the uptake may be reduced in Warthin's tumor mainly with a cystic component. The diagnostic accuracy of salivary gland scintigraphy for Warthin's tumors and oncocytomas is around 90%, but these cannot be differentiated in salivary gland scintigraphy. Because Warthin's tumors develop bilaterally in 5–20% of cases, the contralateral parotid gland should be carefully evaluated. Meanwhile, because 99mTcO4− is not taken up by pleomorphic adenomas or parotid gland cancer (defect images), salivary gland scintigraphy is useful for differentiation [2].

2.5. Kinetic analysis of salivary gland function

The indications for kinetic analysis of salivary gland function include Sjögren's syndrome, acute/chronic sialadenitis, and facial/glossopharyngeal nerve palsy. Salivary gland function is assessed based on dynamic images and TAC. In general, chronic sialadenitis shows a decreased uptake while acute sialadenitis shows an increased uptake; acute/chronic sialadenitis shows a reduced or no response to stimulation of saliva secretion. Uptake in salivary glands is barely evident in patients with severe Sjögren's syndrome (**Figures 6** and **7**). The severity of the reduction in washout after the stimulation of saliva secretion well correlates with the results of the Saxon test. Thus, kinetic analysis reflects the severity of Sjögren's syndrome, allowing an objective assessment of salivary gland function [3].

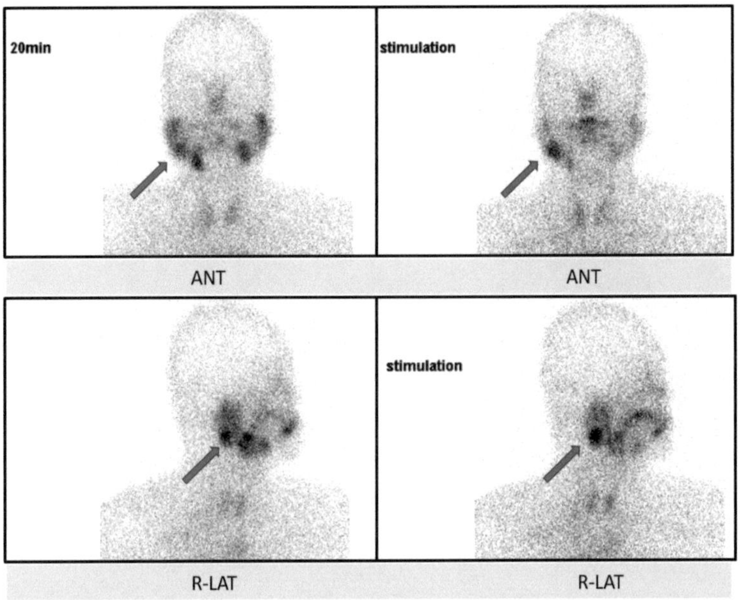

Figure 5. Warthin's tumor. On the image 20 minutes after administration, the radionuclide is taken up by the right parotid gland. After the stimulation of saliva secretion, the radionuclide remains in the right parotid tumor. The diagnosis was Warthin's tumor.

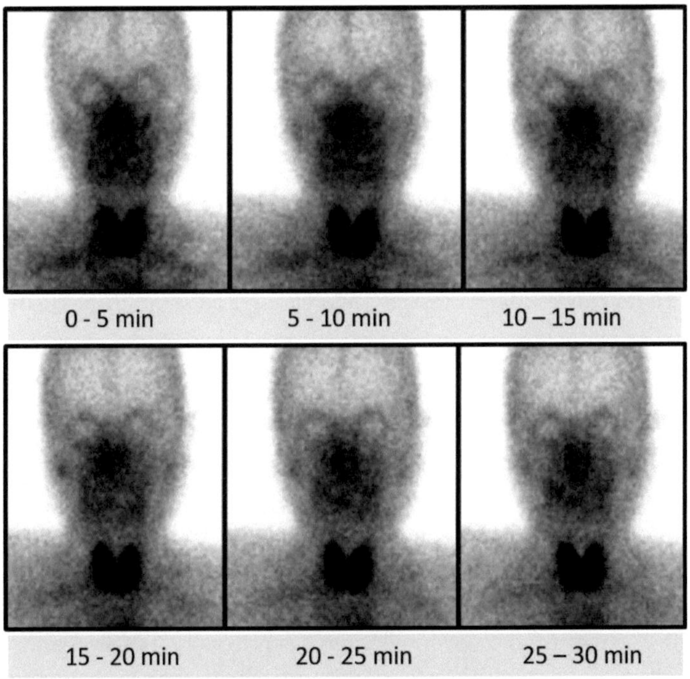

Figure 6. Sjögren's syndrome. All four salivary glands show decreased uptake.

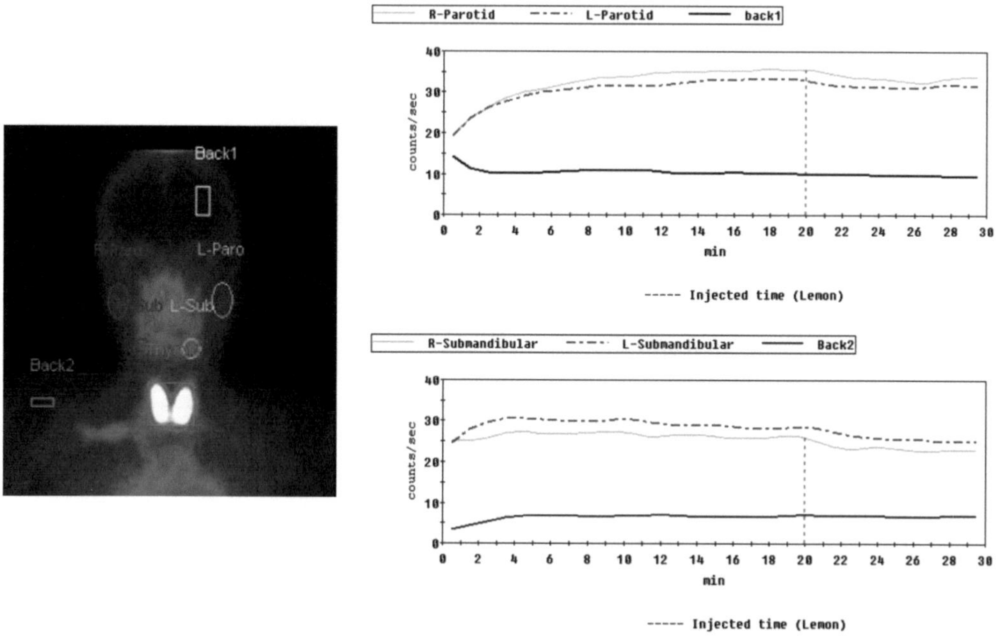

Figure 7. TAC of the Sjögren's syndrome. All four salivary glands show decreased uptake and a poor response to stimulation of saliva secretion 20 minutes after administration. TAC is useful for assessment.

3. Scintigraphy of inflammation (67Ga scintigraphy)

3.1. Mechanism of uptake

67Ga administered intravenously binds to transferrin, a serum protein, and is transported into cells through transferrin receptors. The carbon atom of citrate stabilizes the bond between 67Ga and transferrin. Transferrin receptors that bind to 67Ga distributed in lysosomes and cytoplasm are often present in tumor and inflammatory cells, which show intense uptake of 67Ga.

3.2. Testing procedure and imaging evaluation

67Ga is intravenously administered at a dose of 185–555 MBq. Imaging is performed 48–72 hours after intravenous administration to visualize the distribution of the radionuclide. 67Ga is excreted from the kidney and intestinal tract within 24 hours after administration and is mainly excreted by the liver. Intense uptake of 67Ga is noted in the liver, bone, and spleen 48–72 hours after administration. 67Ga is known to be taken up by inflammation and tumors; however, the sensitivity of 67Ga scintigraphy is low for malignant tumors, while the negative predictive value is high. Thus, a negative finding of focal uptake is likely to represent a benign lesion or low-grade tumor. Focal uptake in the parotid gland on 67Ga scintigraphy is useful for the supplemental diagnosis of Warthin's tumor. Meanwhile, with increased diffuse bilateral uptake, differential diagnosis includes sarcoidosis (**Figure 8**),

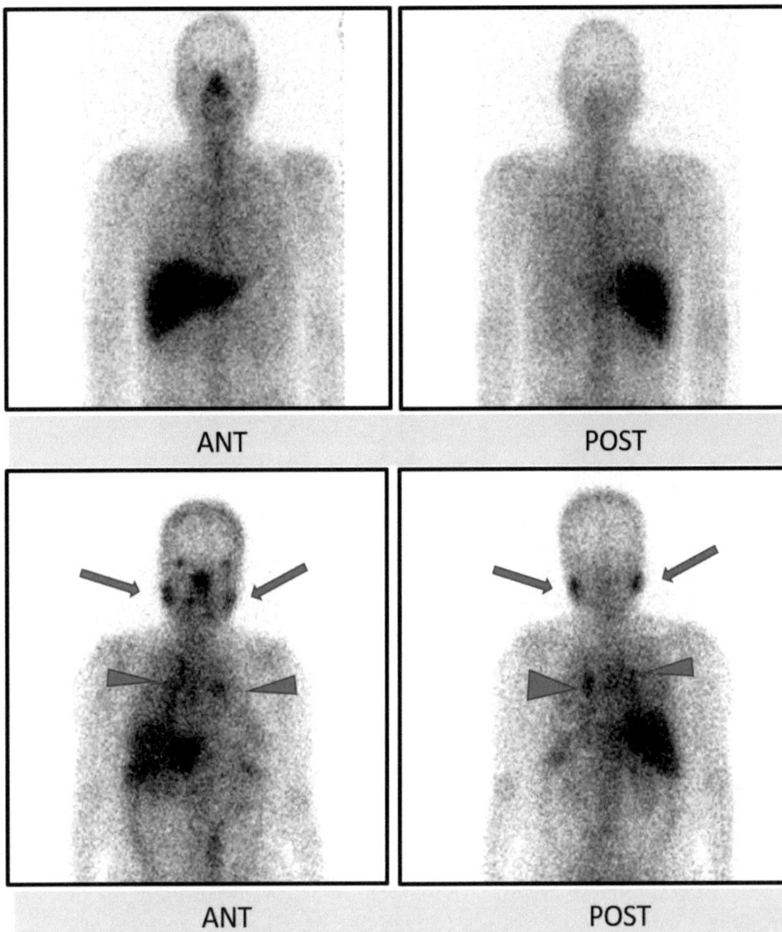

Figure 8. 67Ga scintigraphy. Upper column, normal image; lower column, sarcoidosis. Uptake is noted in the bilateral parotid glands (arrow), and mediastinal/hilar lymph nodes (arrowhead).

IgG4-related disease, Sjögren's syndrome, and Mikulicz disease. In recent years, 67Ga scintigraphy for tumor diagnosis has been increasingly replaced by FDG-PET, as described below.

4. PET

4.1. Mechanism of uptake

FDG-PET is a critical modality for determining the localization, focal lesions, and staging of many malignant tumors, as well as for their follow-up observation. It is also essential for the clinical management of salivary tumors [4–8]. Like glucose, fluorodeoxyglucose (FDG) is taken up by cells via glucose transporters and phosphorylated; however, unlike glucose, FDG remains in cells after phosphorylation. In general, glucose transporters and glucose metabolism are increased in tumor cells, leading to an increased uptake of FDG (**Figure 9**). The widespread use of PET combined with computed tomography (PET/CT) has increased the diagnostic accuracy by compensating for PET disadvantages, including poor spatial resolution and lack of anatomic information. Moreover, PET combined with magnetic resonance imaging (PET/MRI) has recently emerged.

4.2. Testing procedure

Fasting is required for 4 hours before testing and intake of liquids with sugar content is prohibited. FDG (**Figure 10**) is intravenously administered at a dose of 185–444 MBq (5–12 mCi). Imaging is performed 60–90 minutes after administration to visualize distribution. The accumulation is visually and semi-quantitatively assessed using the standardized uptake value (SUV), which is the ratio of uptake to the injected dose per unit body weight.

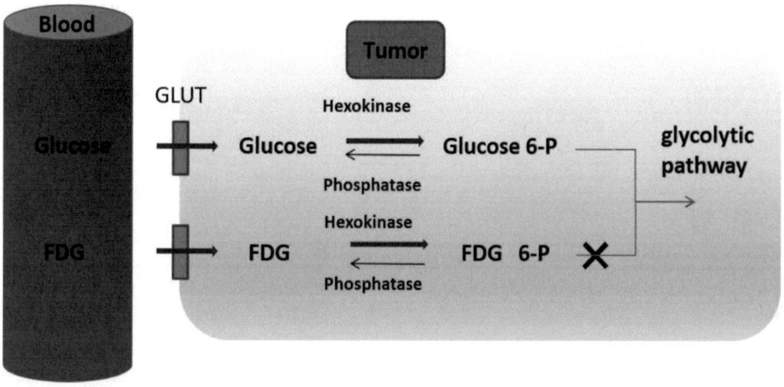

Figure 9. Mechanism of FDG uptake. Like glucose, FDG is taken up by cells via glucose transporters and phosphorylated; however, unlike glucose, FDG remains in cells after phosphorylation.

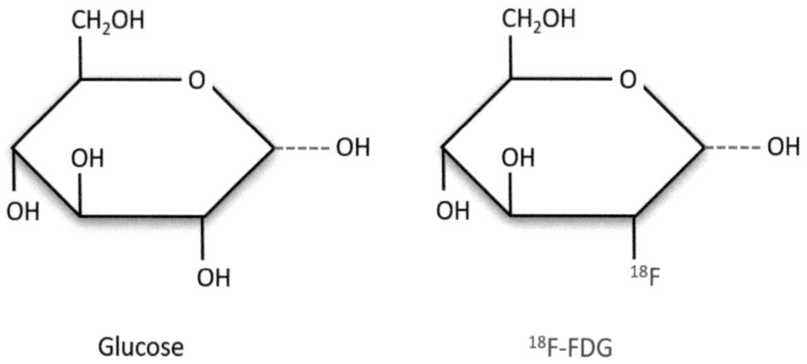

Figure 10. The chemical structure of FDG. The chemical structure of FDG is identical to that of 18F (one of the hydroxy groups of glucose that is replaced by a positron-emitting radionuclide).

4.3. Normal uptake

In the head and neck areas, many structures show physiologic uptake, including salivary glands, nasal and sinonasal mucosa, extraocular muscles, and lymphoid tissue. Because artifacts due to dentures are also often seen, information on CT or MRI images is useful [8].

4.4. Diagnosis of salivary gland tumors

Some lesions are difficult to differentiate from normal structures, postoperative changes, and inflammatory changes on CT or MRI images alone. However, those lesions can be diagnosed through the combined use of FDG-PET [4, 5, 7]. FDG-PET for medical evaluation or staging of a malignant tumor may incidentally reveal a salivary gland tumor [7, 9].

The differentiation of benign from malignant parotid tumors is difficult based on the results of FDG uptake alone. Moreover, the differentiation of benign from malignant salivary tumors is often difficult based on the comparison of the results of SUVmax alone. A malignant tumor tends to show more intense FDG uptake than a benign tumor; however, benign tumors, such as Warthin's tumor and pleomorphic adenoma (**Figure 11**) [10–12], also show high FDG

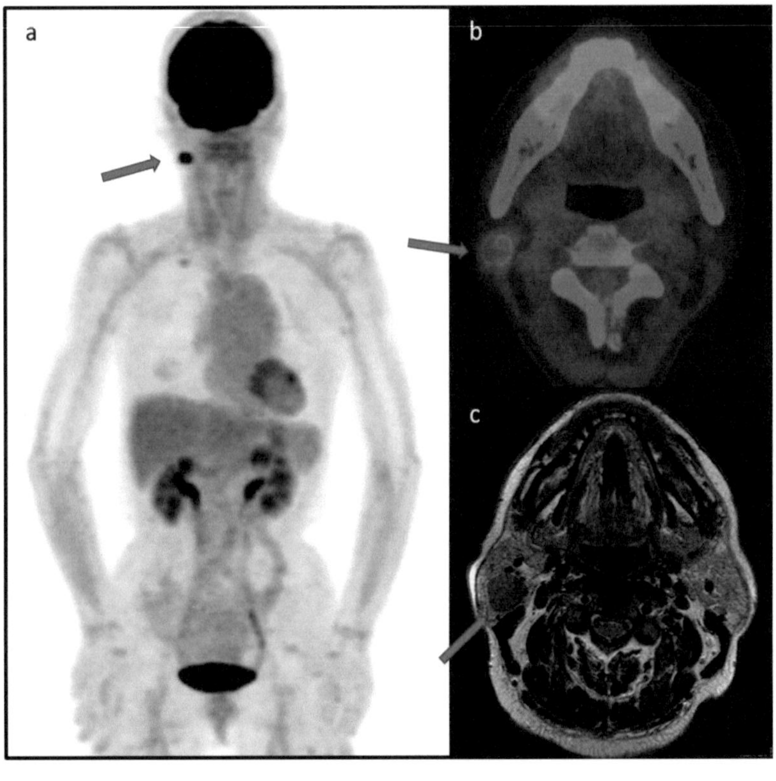

Figure 11. Warthin's tumor. (a). PET MIP image. (b). PET/CT fusion image. (c). T1-weighted MRI image. FDG is strongly taken up by the tumor (SUVmax: 9.4) in the right parotid gland. MRI also provides many findings consistent with malignancy. Salivary gland scintigraphy is useful for differentiation.

uptake. Some studies have reported that the differentiation of benign from malignant salivary tumors is possible with the use of indices such as dual-time-point (DTP) imaging and tumor volume, in addition to SUVmax [4, 5].

The sensitivity of PET/CT is approximately 80% for the detection of preoperative primary lesions (**Figure 12**), but the accuracy for staging may vary. In particular, FDG-PET images often show false-positive results for the diagnosis of cervical lymph nodes.

Sialadenitis may show diffuse, increased uptake. However, some cases may show unilateral uptake due to the distribution of inflammation and may be difficult to differentiate from a tumor.

FDG-PET, which provides information about systemic metabolism, is very useful for detecting primary or recurrent lesions for the determination of treatment strategy in cases with highly-malignant tumors requiring aggressive treatment. FDG-PET aids in detection of local involvement, regional lymph node metastasis, distant metastasis, and dissemination for the clinical staging and restaging. It is also useful in the detection of an incidental

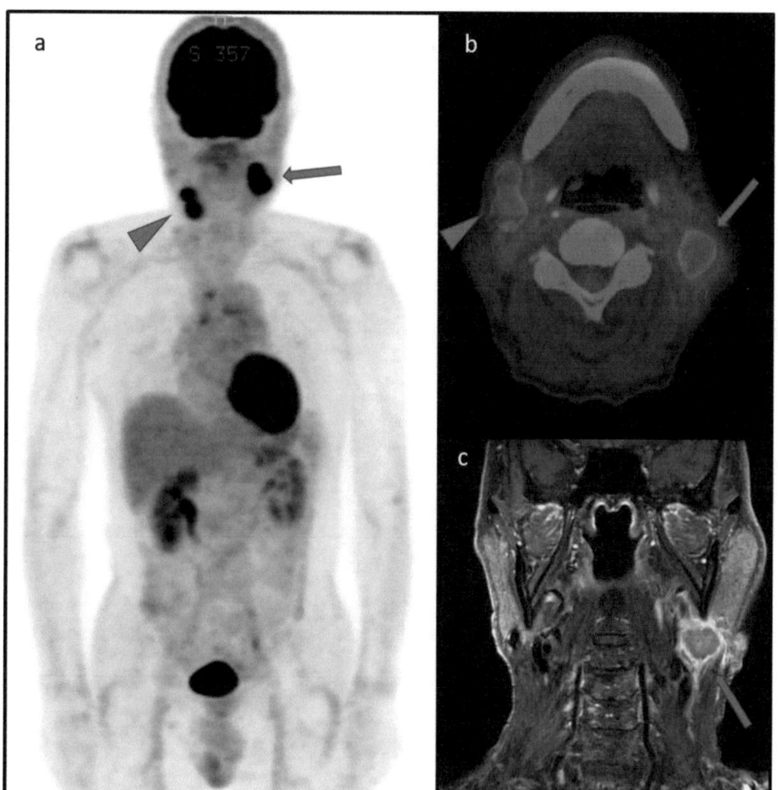

Figure 12. (a). PET MIP image. (b). PET/CT fusion image. (c). T1-weighted MRI using gadolinium-based contrast (GdT1) image. Very strong uptake of FDG (SUVmax: 15.8, arrow) is seen in the region corresponding to the left parotid tumor on the MRI image. Uptake is seen in the region of the right internal jugular lymph nodes (SUVmax: 10.2, arrow head). Parotid cancer or cervical lymph node metastasis is suspected.

cancer. Therefore, this imaging modality is essential before the initiation of treatment and for patient follow-up [4, 5, 13–15].

5. Salivary gland disorders associated with radioiodine therapy

Radioactive iodine (RAI) therapy is the most widely used treatment for differentiated thyroid cancer and has a long history. Because NIS is expressed in the salivary glands, 131I is also incorporated into the salivary glands. Not only thyroid cancer but also salivary glands are irradiated; and thus, acute/chronic sialadenitis may develop.

5.1. Acute salivary gland disorders

Sialadenitis is one of the most common adverse reactions to RAI therapy. Acute-phase sialadenitis causes swelling of the major salivary glands and pain (especially while eating) within one to a few days after oral administration of 131I. Although sialadenitis ameliorates without treatment, xerostomia may develop during the chronic phase and significantly impair the quality of life. Thus, when symptoms develop, sialadenitis should be treated immediately [16, 17]. The parotid glands may be affected more often than the submandibular glands. Steroids are more effective than nonsteroidal anti-inflammatory drugs. Cooling and frequent rinsing with cold water may relieve symptoms. Taste dysfunction is characterized by reduced acuity for salt taste and subsequently sweet taste; bitter taste remains unaffected. Taste dysfunction may become obvious later (2–4 weeks after 131I administration), rather than immediately after administration. To prevent an acute-phase disorder, snacks such as lemon candy to stimulate saliva secretion may be helpful because they also promote the excretion of 131I. Apitherapy using honey products is reportedly useful for preventing salivary gland disorders. Massage of the salivary glands and aroma therapy are also reported to relieve symptoms [18].

5.2. Chronic salivary gland disorders

Xerostomia may develop during the chronic phase, even in patients without acute impairment. Permanent dysfunction is reported to develop more frequently in the submandibular glands than in the parotid glands. Salivary gland scintigraphy shows a pattern of obstructive dysfunction before revealing parenchymal damage of the salivary gland. Therefore, salivary gland function may improve if salivary gland dysfunction can be identified within the period showing an obstructive pattern [19]. Salivary gland function should be monitored regularly with scintigraphy or other studies [20].

6. Conclusions

Radionuclide imaging of salivary glands has been used not only for functional assessment but also for comprehensive diagnosis including morphological information with the advent of single-photon emission computed tomography (SPECT)/CT and PET/CT. Although scientific

http://dx.doi.org/10.5772/intechopen.70622

evidence is limited, the advantages of radionuclide scanning should be determined. For RAI therapy, attention should be paid to adverse reactions. Coordination among healthcare providers including nurses, radiological technologists, and doctors of all departments involved in treatment is important for achieving effective outcomes.

Acknowledgements

This work was supported by JSPS KAKENHI Grant Number 16K20745.

Author details

Michihiro Nakayama*, Atsutaka Okizaki, Kaori Nakajima and Koji Takahashi

*Address all correspondence to: m-naka@asahikawa-med.ac.jp

Department of Radiology, Asahikawa Medical University, Japan

References

[1] Pilbrow W, et al. Salivary gland scintigraphy–A suitable substitute for sialography? The British Journal of Radiology. 1990;**63**:190-196

[2] Miyake H, et al. Warthin's tumor of parotid gland on Tc-99m pertechnetate scintigraphy with lemon juice stimulation: Tc-99m uptake, size, and pathologic correlation. European Radiology. 2001;**11**:2472-2478

[3] Shizukuishi K, et al. Gland scintigraphy in patients with Sjogren's syndrome. Annals of Nuclear Medicine. 2003;**17**:627-631

[4] Jeong HS, et al. Role of 18 F-FDG PET/CT in management of high-grade salivary gland malignancies. Nuclear-Medizin. 2007;**48**:1237-1244

[5] Nakayama M, et al. Dual-time-point F-18 FDG PET/CT imaging for differentiating the lymph nodes between malignant lymphoma and benign lesions. Annals of Nuclear Medicine. 2013;**27**:163-169. DOI: 10.1007/s12149-012-0669-1

[6] Hadiprodjo D, et al. Parotid gland tumors: Preliminary data for the value of FDG PET/CT diagnostic parameters. AJR. American Journal of Roentgenology. 2012;**198**:W185-W190

[7] Wang HC, et al. Efficacy of conventional whole-body 18F-FDG PET/CT in the incidental findings of parotid masses. Annals of Nuclear Medicine. 2010;**24**:571-577

[8] Blodgett TM, et al. Combined PET-CT in the head and neck: Part 1. Physiologic. Altered physiologic, and artifactual FDG uptake. Radiographies. 2005;**25**:897-912

[9] Lee SK, et al. Parotid incidentaloma identified by combined 18F-fluorodeoxyglucose whole-body positron emission tomography and computed tomography: Findings at grayscale and power Doppler ultrasonography and ultrasound-guided fine-needle aspiration biopsy or core-needle biopsy. European Radiology. 2009;**19**:2268-2274

[10] McGuirt WF, et al. Preoperative identification of benign vs. malignant parotid masses: A comparative study including positron emission tomography. Laryngoscope. 1995;**105**: 579-584

[11] Keyes JW Jr, et al. Salivary gland tumors: Pretherapy evaluation with PET. Radiology 1994;**192**:99-102

[12] Uchida Y, et al. Diagnostic value of FDG PET and salivary gland scintigraphy for parotid tumors. Clinical Nuclear Medicine. 2005;**30**:170-176

[13] Kim KH, et al. The significance of CT scan or MRI in the evaluation of salivary gland tumors. Auris Nasus Larynx. 1998;**25**:397-402

[14] Otsuka H, et al. The impact of FDG-PET in the management of patients with salivary gland malignancy. Annals of Nuclear Medicine. 2005;**19**:691-694

[15] Rob JL, et al. Clinical utility of 18F-FDG PET for patients with salivary gland malignancies. Journal of Nuclear Medicine. 2007;**48**:240-246

[16] Alexander C, Bader JB, Schaefer A, Finke C, Kirsch CM. Intermediate and long-term side effects of high-dose radioiodine therapy for thyroid carcinoma. Journal of Nuclear Medicine. 1998;**39**:1551-1554

[17] Lee SL. Complications of radioactive iodine treatment of thyroid carcinoma. Journal of the National Comprehensive Cancer Network. 2010;**8**:1277-1286

[18] Nakayama M, et al. A randomized controlled trial for the effectiveness of aromatherapy in decreasing salivary gland damage following radioactive iodine therapy for differentiated thyroid cancer. BioMed Research International. 2016;**2016**, Article ID 9509810:6. DOI: 10.1155/2016/9509810

[19] Kim YM, et al. Salivary gland function after sialendoscopy for treatment of chronic radioiodine-induced sialadenitis. Head & Neck. 2016;**38**:51-58

[20] Jeong SY, et al. Salivary gland function 5 years after radioactive iodine ablation in patients with differentiated thyroid cancer: Direct comparison of pre- and postablation scintigraphies and their relation to xerostomia symptoms. Thyroid. 2013;**23**:609-616

Section 3

New Approaches in the Treatment of Salivary Gland Diseases

Chapter 7

Salivary Effects of Facial Vibrotactile Stimulation in Patients with Sjogren's Syndrome and Poor Salivation

Koichiro Ueda, Kanako Gora, Masaru Yamaoka, Takako Sato, Kimiko Abe, Enri Nakayama, Mituyasu Sato, Yumiko Tunoda, Sumiko Akatuka, Sayaka Fukui, Akinari Hayashi, Teruyuki Hirai, Sayako Ohnishi, Mayumi Hayata and Hisao Hiraba

Additional information is available at the end of the chapter

http://dx.doi.org/10.5772/intechopen.72383

Abstract

We examined the effect of vibrotactile apparatus in patients with Sjögren's syndrome and others with reduced salivation in comparison to normal subjects. The most effective salivation in normal subjects was produced by 89 Hz vibrotactile stimulation with 9.8 μm amplitude on the parotid or submandibular glands vibrotactile stimuli. First, we examined by measuring the weight of dental cotton rolls positioned at the opening of the secretory duct for total salivation 3 min during resting, and then after 5-min intervals, *the weights were measured every 3 min* of vibrotactile stimulation on salivary glands. Furthermore, we measured facial temperature around vibrators after 2 min of vibration. We investigated 10 poor salivation patients with Sjögren's syndrome (8 patients) defined by examinations (contrast study or scintigraphic test) and others (2 patients). About 50% of patients with poor salivation gained recognition for good results, although they had periods of short-term (3 months) and long-term effects (6–7 years) during recuperation. Furthermore, *facial skin temperatures on both sides of parotid glands were decreased in Sjogren's syndrome after vibration, although their temperatures were increased following recovery.* Although the mechanism is not clear, we think that vibrotactile stimulation gives activation to salivary glands under the rising facial temperature.

Keywords: vibrotactile stimulation, facial skin temperature, parotid and submandibular glands, poor salivation, Sjögren's syndrome

1. Introduction

When we treat patients with reduced salivation (hyposalivation), we provide treatments such as artificial saliva, humectant, massage on the salivary glands, and so on [1]. However, treatment *with* the artificial saliva and humectant is the symptomatic treatment, and patients with handicaps *experience difficulties when they do massage*. We previously reported about *the* relationship between facial vibratory effects in normal subjects and promotion of salivation. *We performed this method* for facial vibratory effects *on* Sjögren's syndrome patients with poor salivation. We focused *on increase of* salivation with the use of facial vibrotactile stimulation, as reported by Hiraba et al. [2, 9, 10].

When patients continuously utilize the apparatus in future *the decrease or increase of salivation is examined from this result* [3]. *In this experiment*, it was necessary to make a comparison between the resting and *stimulated* salivations and to investigate the most effective frequency for increasing the salivary secretion. We examined the amount of salivation during vibrotactile stimuli with one vibrating motor (1.9 μm amplitude) on the bilateral masseter muscle belly (on the parotid glands), and in patients of Sjögren's syndrome, we asked twice practice during 15 min of morning and night. Furthermore, *the* amount of salivation *was* explored by using a dental cotton roll positioned at the opening of the secretory duct for 3 *min*. After this experiment was performed, *we made* a comparison between the resting and *stimulated* salivations and *investigated* the most effective frequency for increasing salivary secretion. *When we examined normal subjects, the effect of the increased salivation determined the difference between the resting and stimulated salivations. We think that total salivation after the resting phase shows conditions of day-to-day salivation, and they after the stimulating are effects of vibrotactile stimulation.*

We defined 5-min intervals as the recovery time between the resting and *stimulated* salivations from the previous pre-examinations. Furthermore, we examined temperature effects *on* patients with poor salivations (affected by Sjogren's syndrome) and others by the use of facial vibrotactile stimuli. Increased facial temperature by the vibrotactile stimulation showed changes of metabolism around facial skins. We will discuss the effects of vibrotactile stimulation based on these results.

2. Material and methods

2.1. Vibrotactile stimulation apparatus

The vibrotactile stimulation apparatus consists of an oscillating body and control unit, as shown in **Figure 1A** [2]. The oscillating body is composed of the headset equipped with vibrators as a substitute for positions of the bilateral microphones and vibrators utilizing the vibration electric motor (VEM) (Rekishin Japan Co., LE12AOG), as shown in **Figure 1A**. The VEM *is* covered in silicon rubber (polyethyl methacrylate, dental mucosa protective material, Shyofu Co.) for conglobating the parts under stimulation and preventing the warming of the VEM's temperature produced by the vibration of long periods [2]. The control unit consists

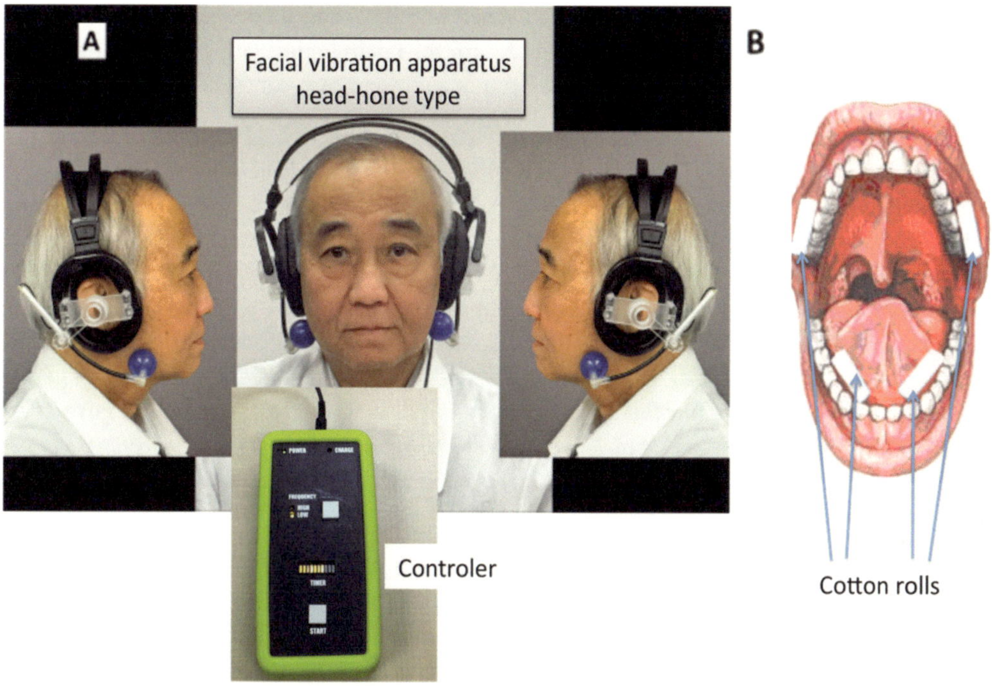

Figure 1. (A) Apparatus for facial vibration and (B) position of cotton rolls.

of three parts: the pulse width modulation (PWM) circuit, LCD monitor circuit and power supply circuit, and *interfaces* with a PWN electric motor, *delivers* vibration frequencies in the 60–182 Hz range [4].

As shown in **Figure 1**, we examined the amount of salivation during vibrotactile stimuli by two kinds of methods: on the bilateral masseter muscles belly (parotid glands) and on the bilateral parts of submandibular angle (submandibular glands). We examined the amount of salivation using a dental cotton roll (1 cm across and 3 cm length) positioned at the opening of the secretory ducts (right and left sides of parotid glands and right and left sides of submandibular and sublingual glands), during the vibrotactile stimuli on the bilateral parotid and submandibular glands, and wet cotton rolls measured for 3 min. These weights were then compared to their initiatory weights, as shown in **Figure 1B** [2].

2.2. Estimation of the stimulating salivation in normal subjects

First, we use three different frequencies, 89, 114 and 180 Hz as the vibrotactile frequency from the character of the oscillating body on the parotid glands. **Figure 1** *shows the apparatus and position of rolls. To begin with, we put an exercise into practice for avoiding foreign-body sensation on the cotton rolls while setting for 3 min.* Next, after 5 min of *resting*, we examined the amount of salivation during the 89 Hz vibrotactile stimulation for 3 min. *Furthermore, after every 5 min of rest, we examined next amount of salivation during the 114 and 180 Hz vibrotactile stimuli for 3 min, respectively.* We decided on 3 min *for* the measurement *of* salivation and 5 min *for* recovery time from the previous experiment [2]. We carried out the examinations and used 19 normal subjects (male: 6 and female: 13, average age 22) for the resting-stimulating examination. This experiment was performed between 3 and 5 pm in a temperature-controlled room.

Second, as shown in **Figure 2**, *we used three different frequencies (89, 114 and 180 Hz) and two different amplitudes (1.9 and 3.5 μm) on the parotid and/or submandibular glands. Amplitudes of vibrotactile stimuli were measured by the CCD laser displacement gauge (LK-G3000, KEYENCE Co.). After three different frequencies were attempted on the parotid glands, we explored the most effective frequency, and we arrived at a frequency of 89 Hz. We examined the frequency of 89 and 114 Hz and we used also oscillating bodies added as the frequency with double motors (one motor is 1.9 μm amplitude and double motors is 3.5 μm amplitude). Namely, the second experiment was practiced by 89 and 114 Hz with one motors (1.9 μm amplitude), and 89 and 114 Hz with double motors (3.5 μm amplitude). We examined the amount of salivation in four different trials, as shown in* **Figure 2**. *We carried out the examinations and used 17 normal subjects (male: 15 and female: 2, average age: 22) for the resting-stimulating examination. This experiment was performed between 3 and 5 pm in a temperature-controlled room.*

Finally, as shown in **Figure 2**, since the most effective salivation by vibrotactile stimuli was at 89 Hz frequency with one motor (1.9 μm amplitude), we examined salivations on 89 Hz vibrotactile stimulation *continuously for* 4 or 5 days. *As patients continuously utilized the apparatus, we examined if adaptation develops with everyday usage and whether or not the decrease of salivation arises.* We investigated the adaptation of periods with the continuous use of vibrotactile stimuli for 4 continuous days in the same subjects. We carried out *this examination* and used 26

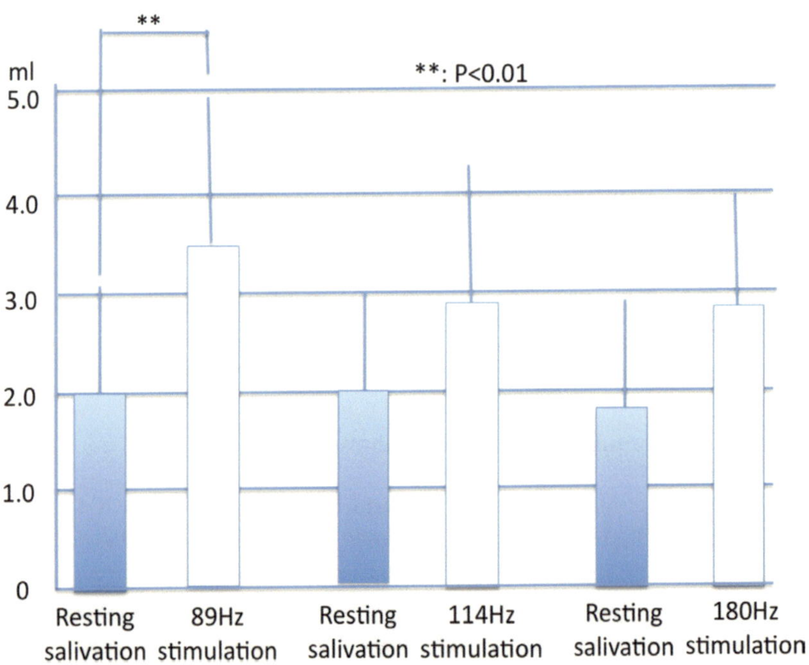

Figure 2. Salivations in each vibration frequency.

normal subjects (male: 11 and female: 15, average age 25) for the resting-stimulating examination. This experiment was performed between 3 and 5 pm in a temperature-controlled room. *In particular, we find that 89 Hz frequency and 1.9 μm amplitude is most effective for salivation.*

2.3. Vibrotactile stimuli on the parotid and submandibular glands

As shown in **Figure 1**, we examined the difference between vibrotactile stimuli on the parotid glands and the submandibular glands. First, we tried three different vibrotactile stimuli, 89, 114, and 180 Hz, on the parotid glands and explored the frequency for the most effective salivation, as shown in **Figure 2**. Next, we inferred the most effective salivation of 89 Hz with the one motor depending on vibrotactile stimuli on the parotid or submandibular glands [2]. Furthermore, we investigated the most effective salivation depending on the difference of amplitudes (1.9 and 3.5 μm amplitudes). We inferred the most effective salivation of 89 Hz with the one motor (1.9 microm amplitude) on the submandibular glands (significant difference $P < 0.05$, 89 Hz with 1.9 μm amplitude and 114 Hz with 1.9 and 3.5 μm amplitude), as shown in Hiraba et al. [2].

2.4. Total salivation after the vibrotactile stimulation on the parotid or submandibular and sublingual glands

In 89 Hz vibrotactile stimulation with 1.9 μm amplitude on the parotid glands, we observed the most effective salivation in each gland, the right parotid, left parotid, right submandibular and sublingual, and left submandibular and sublingual glands. *Vibrotactile stimuli on the parotid or submandibular glands in any case showed that at 89 Hz more effective salivation in the right and left parotid and in the left and right submandibular and sublingual glands happened in comparison with the resting salivation in each gland.* On the other hand, vibrotactile stimuli with 1.9 μm (89 and 114 Hz—1) or 3.5 μm amplitudes (89 and 114 Hz—2) on the parotid or submandibular glands were examined. The 89 Hz with one motor, was the most effective salivation in the parotid, and the submandibular and sublingual glands, and the 89 Hz with double motors, was the more effective salivation in the parotid, and submandibular and sublingual glands, as shown in Hiraba et al. [2]. From these reasons, we suggested that vibrotactile stimulation at 89 Hz with 1.9 μm amplitude showed the most effective salivation in many glands.

Finally, we assumed that 89 Hz with 1.9 μm amplitude vibrotactile stimulation *produced the most effective salivation,* and then the vibrotactile stimuli on the parotid and submandibular glands *showed* hardly any difference. We then decided to use the apparatus to patients affected by poor salivation.

2.5. Information of patients with poor salivation affected by Sjögren's syndrome and others

In **Figure 3**, we showed information of patients: eight women were *diagnosed with* Sjögren's syndrome and two women's symptoms were unexplained. *Patients with Sjögren's syndrome were diagnosed by contrast and/or scintigraphic studies. In particular, the patients with indefinite complaints were not given a definite diagnosis; nevertheless, they had poor salivation as their chief complaint.*

Name	Definite diagnosis	Saligren Dose level	Passed years	Actual condition
1. MZ	contrast study	dispense medication (3 drugs/day)	8 years	continued investigation
2. AS	contrast study	dispense medication (3 drugs/day)	5 years	break up for myalgia
3. NI	contrast & scintigraphic study	dispense medication (3 drugs/day)	5 years	vibration disamenity
4. KM	contrast study	dispense medication (3 drugs/day)	3 years	ope of brain cancer
5. TO	scintigraphic study	dispense medication (3 drugs/day)	6 years	contiuued investigation
6. YA	contrast & scintigraphic study	dispense medication (3 drugs/day)	1.5years	cured patient
7. NA	scintigraphic study	no drug	6 years	continued investigation
8. UJ	indefinite complaint	no drug	4 years	break up for change residence
9. SG	indefinite complaint	dispense medication (3 drugs/day)	2 years	ope of brain cancer
10. KN	contrast study	dispense medication (3 drugs/day)	3 years	vibration disamenity

Figure 3. Information of subjects. Patients in 8 and 9 showed only poor salivation. Others are Sjögren's syndrome patients.

3. Results

3.1. Variation per day of the effective salivation on the continuous vibrotactile stimulation

We examined whether or not the effective salivation occurred continuously when the vibrotactile stimulation was carried out every day. Normal subjects (26, males 15 and females 11, average age 25) used this apparatus continuously 4 or 5 days *at* the same time and place [8]. Since patients with *decreased* salivation (hyposalivation) had the psychiatric disorder in daily life, we conducted the experiment to realistically approximate the natural condition. In particular, we produced the analysis following the 89 Hz vibrotactile stimulation with 1.9 μm amplitude from the previous experiment, because this frequency produced the most effective salivation. *No gland (right and left parotid glands, and right submandibular and sublingual glands) showed a decreasing tendency with use day after day* [8].

3.2. Facial skin temperature and heart rate in normal subjects

As shown in **Figure 4A**, facial temperature under vibration apparatus was increased about 0.5°C in 2 or 3 min, and then after 15 min of *continuous stimulation,* it was up by about 0.5°C, too. *Namely, a rise in facial temperature and an increase in RR intervals (decreasing heart rate) by vibration were affected by period of stimulating time. On the other hand, by raising about 200 ms of RR intervals after 15 min an increase in heart rate was observed when the vibration was over. The reason was thought to be parasympathetic activation recoil by vibration stimulation.*

http://dx.doi.org/10.5772/intechopen.72383

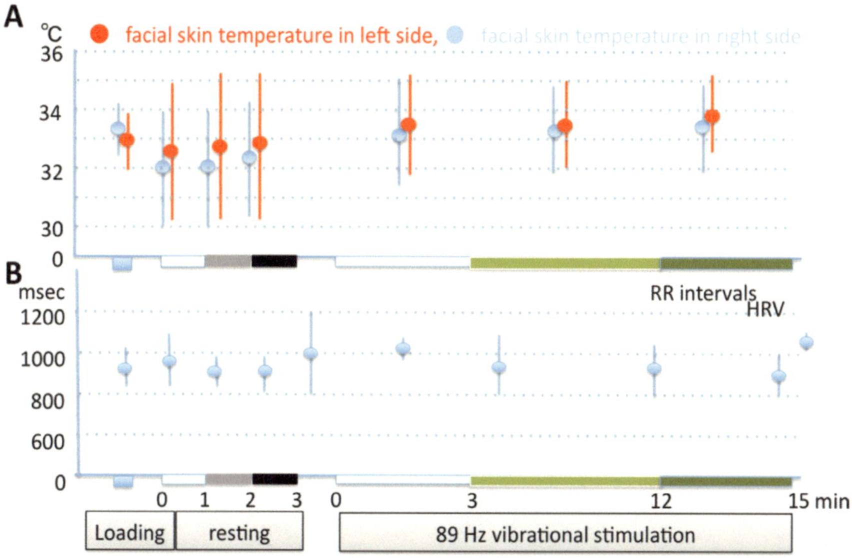

Figure 4. Facial skin temperature (A) and heart rate (B) in normal subjects.

3.3. The relationships between affected and unaffected patients after the vibrotactile stimulation

In **Figure 5A**, we showed changes to saliva production (**Figure 5A-a**) and facial temperature (**Figure 5A-b**) in the *patients who were affected* followed the vibrotactile stimulation. On the other hand, in **Figure 5B**, we showed changes to saliva production (**Figure 5B-a**) and facial temperature (**Figure 5B-b**) in *patients who were not affected* followed the vibrotactile stimulation. As shown in **Figure 5A**, the saliva production (elevated state from avg. 0.2 to 1.5 ml) was exponentially increased after about 5 years. The finding was shown as changes to increased face temperature (in a positive direction). However, as shown in **Figure 5B**, the saliva production and facial temperature remained static.

3.4. *The affected and unaffected* patients on the vibrotactile stimulation

In **Figures 5** and **6**, *affected* patients were divided into apocatastasis for a long period and for a short period. *Affected* patients with a long period were exponentially increased after about 6 (A), 5 (B) and 1.5 (D) years. Ones with a short period were exponentially increased after about 2 months (E). Facial temperature was increased *with* increased saliva production. On the other hand, in **Figure 7**, *in unaffected patients, the saliva production* and facial temperature remained static.

3.5. Questionnaire data

In **Figure 8**, we showed a survey and patients with satisfaction (good) or non-satisfaction (no/yes or bad) were examined. Patients with satisfaction had many good tendencies, but ones with non-satisfaction had many no/yes and bad.

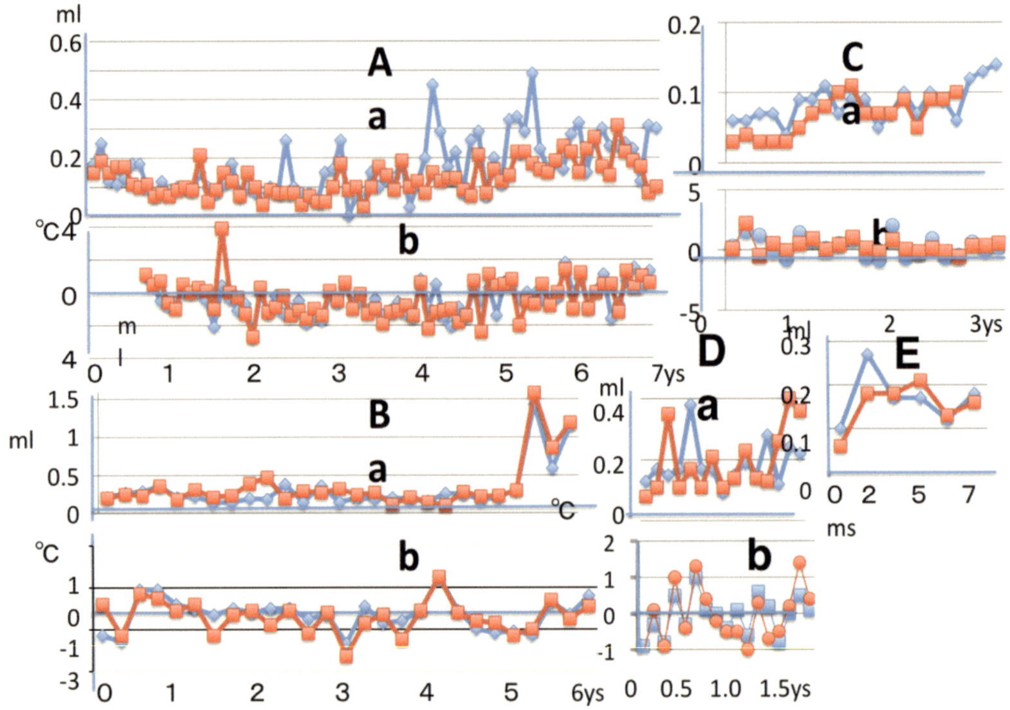

Figure 5. *Patients affected* by a facial vibration. A: salivation gradually increased, and temperature changed to plus tendency near 7 years. On the other hand, patients in B rapidly increased, and temperature changed to plus tendency near 6 years. Patients in C, D and E gradually increased.

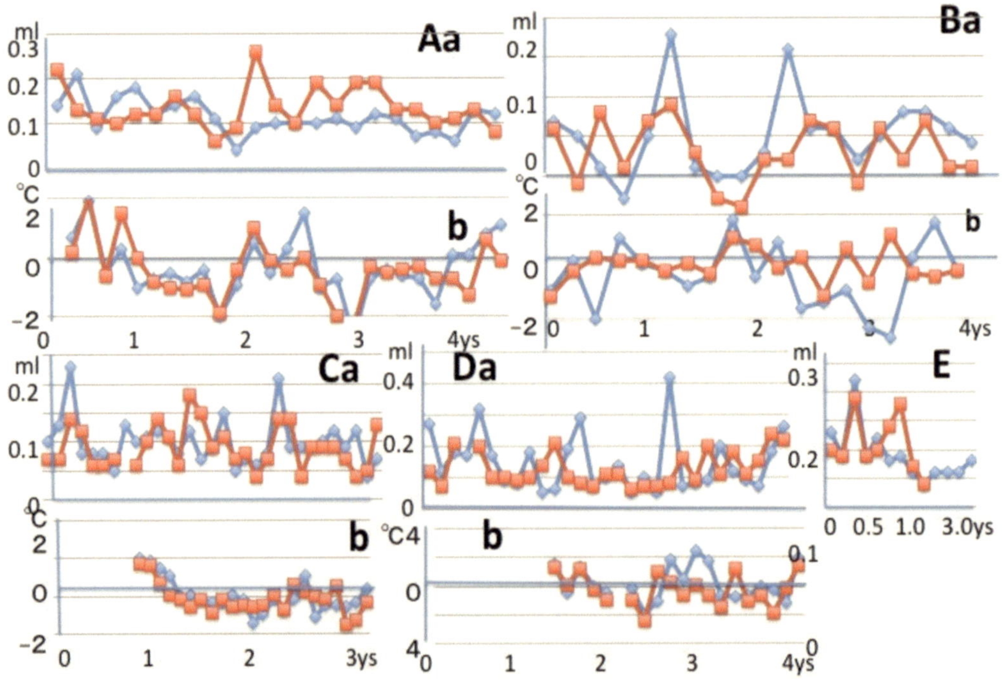

Figure 6. *Patients unaffected* by a facial vibration.

http://dx.doi.org/10.5772/intechopen.72383

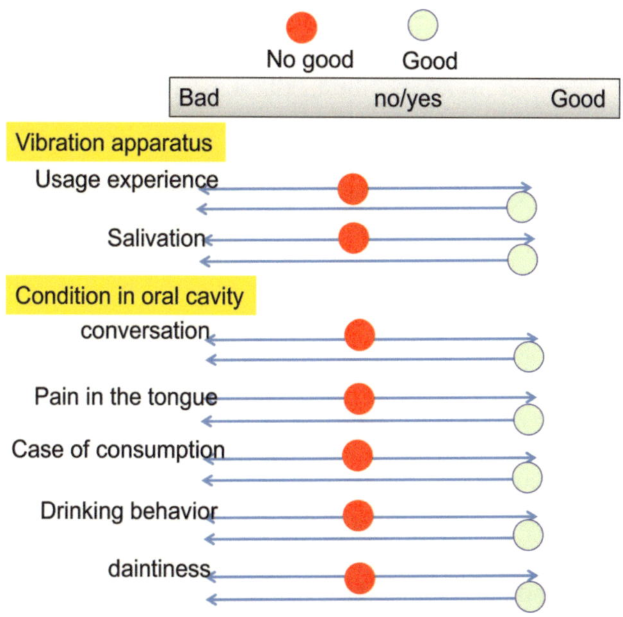

Figure 7. Typical examples of questionnaire data. We divided into three types (bad, no/yes and good) during effects of vibration apparatus and condition in oral cavity after vibration. Effect example is good (blue circles), and no-effect one is no/yes (red circles).

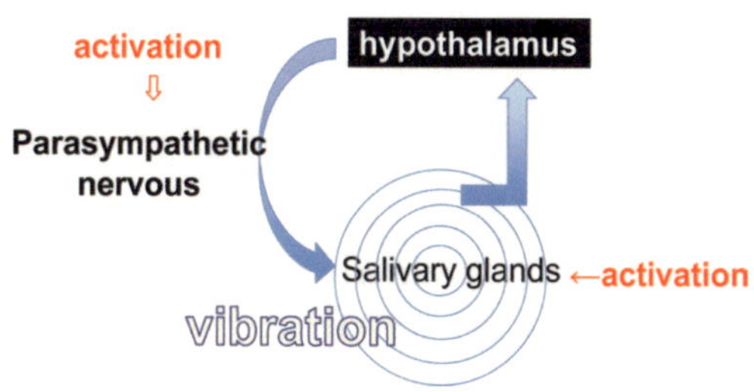

Figure 8. Summary of vibration effects. Facial vibration produces revitalization of cells of salivary glands. Furthermore, stimulation of vibration is activated at hypothalamus, and parasympathetic nerve is activated again. In particular, double activation shows 89 Hz frequency and 1.9 μm amplitude is the most effective vibration.

4. Discussion

The continuous use of various sensory stimuli has been known to induce an adaptation [3, 7]. So we examined *the effects of vibrotactile stimulation and the adaptation in normal subjects, when the patients* continuously used this apparatus every day. *The patients' first desire is not to have an increase in salivary secretion from all salivary glands. However, the increase of total secretion quantities is necessary.* So, we first investigated changes in the total secretion quantities of normal subjects with the vibrotactile stimulation using a cotton roll indwelling each duct of each gland.

On parotid glands, 89 Hz vibrotactile stimuli were shown *to result in* the more effective salivation in the right and left parotid glands and submandibular and sublingual glands, as shown in **Figure 2**. On the other hand, on the submandibular glands, 89 Hz vibrotactile stimuli with one motor were shown *to result in* the more effective salivation in all the glands. The findings suggest the 89 Hz vibrotactile stimuli with one motor may be the most effective salivation, and glands stimulated by vibrotactile stimuli have the tendency *for* the most effective salivation. Namely, on the parotid gland and on the submandibular gland vibrotactile stimuli shows the submandibular and sublingual gland, the place of stimulating portions may be the body of the mandible.

Burdette and Gale studied the effects of treatments in myofascial pain dysfunction patients [5]. Furthermore, Vrjama and Vanharantra [6] reported that discographically painful discs always produced painless feeling in the vibration examination. These facts assume that peripheral stimuli provided by vibration arrive at the central nerve (in the spinal cord and brain stem) and that these effects were exercised by the depressant effect in the cerebral cortex depending on the somatosensory information. Namely, we think that the vibration stimuli may promote the parasympathetic effects by the inhibition of sympathetic effects elicited by the pain, and so on. On the other hand, we know that the production of salivation only induces the parasympathetic effects. Furthermore, the production of salivation will be at a specific frequency and amplitude. This phenomenon may be directly produced by the vibrotactile stimulation of 89 Hz with one motor on the parotid and submandibular glands.

On the other hand, we *examined t*he physiological characteristics of the adaptation to the vibrotactile stimulation, whether *it caused decreased salivation or not. A continuous examination was performed for 4 or 5 days on* 26 normal subjects [8]. Since patients with the *decreased* salivation (hyposalivation) are not exclusively happy in every day of their daily life, we conducted the experiment to realistically approximate the natural conditions. *We did not show decreased adaptation* depending on the continuous using of this apparatus, as shown in **Figure 4**. The result suggests that 89 Hz vibrotactile stimulation of the facial skin on the masseter belly may be appropriate for patients with the *decreased* salivation. Furthermore, we imagined mechanism of salivary production following facial vibration in **Figure 8**. Facial vibration directly activates the poor salivation of grands and then it indirectly parasympathetic nerve via hypothalamus.

Acknowledgements

The authors are grateful to Professor C.S. Langham for carefully reading and editing the manuscript. This work was supported by Sato and Sogoshigaku research grant of Nihon University School of Dentistry, by Grants-in-Aid for Scientific Research (21592539) and by a grant from the Ministry of Education, Culture, Sports, Science, and Technology to promote multidisciplinary research projects.

Appendices and nomenclatures

Obey neuroscience society.

http://dx.doi.org/10.5772/intechopen.72383

Author details

Koichiro Ueda[1], Kanako Gora[1], Masaru Yamaoka[2], Takako Sato[3], Kimiko Abe[1], Enri Nakayama[1], Mituyasu Sato[1], Yumiko Tunoda[4], Sumiko Akatuka[4], Sayaka Fukui[4], Akinari Hayashi[1], Teruyuki Hirai[1], Sayako Ohnishi[1], Mayumi Hayata[1] and Hisao Hiraba[1]*

*Address all correspondence to: hiraba.hisao@nihon-u.ac.jp

1 Department of Dysphasia Rehabilitation, Nihon University, School of Dentistry, Tokyo, Japan

2 Department of Basic Science, Nihon University, School of Dentistry, Tokyo, Japan

3 Department of Oral Surgery, Nihon University, School of Dentistry, Tokyo, Japan

4 Department of Dental Hospital at Surugadai, Nihon University, School of Dentistry, Tokyo, Japan

References

[1] Ueda K. IV-2 Sessyoku enge rehabilitation. In: Uematsu H, Inaba S, Watanabe M, editors. Koureishya Shika Guidebook. Tokyo: Ishiyaku; 2005. pp. 248-275. (in Japanese)

[2] Hiraba H, Yamaoka M, Fukano M, Ueda K, Fujiwara T. Increased secretion of salivary glands produced by facial vibrotactile stimulation. Somatosensory and Motor Research. 2008;**25**:222-229

[3] Despopoulos A, Silbernagl S. 10 Nutrion and digeston. In: Color Atlas of Physiology. 5th ed. New York: Medical Science International Ltd.; 2003. pp. 226-265

[4] Yamaoka M, Hiraba H, Ueda K, Fujiwara T. Development of a vibratile stimulation apparatus for orofacial rehabilitation. Nihondaigaku Shigakubu Kiyou. 2007;**35**:13-18. (in Japanese)

[5] Burdette BH, Gale EN. The effects of treatment on masticatory muscle activity and mandibular posture in myofascial pain-dysfunction patients. Journal of Dental Research. 1986;**67**:1126-1130

[6] Vriama M, Vanharanta H. Bony vibrotactail stimulation: A new, non-invasive method for examining intradiscal pain. European Spine Journal. 1994;**3**:233-235

[7] Desmedt JE, Codaux E. Vibration induced discharge patterns of single motor unit in the masseter muscle in man. The Journal of Physiology. 1975;**253**:420-442

[8] Hiraba H, Sato T, Nishimura S, Yamaoka M, Inoue M, Sato M, Iida T, Wada S, Fujiwara T, Ueda K. Chapter 16: Changes in brain blood flow on frontal cortex depending on facial vibrotactile stimuli. In: Vibration Analysis and Control-New Trends and Developments. Francisco Beltran-Carbajal edite. Croatia: InTech; 2011. pp. 337-352. http://www.intech-web.org

[9] Hiraba H, Inoue M, Sato T, Nishimura S, Yamaoka M, Shimano T, Sampei R, Ebihara K, Ishii H, Ueda K. Chapter 14: Optimal vibrotactile stimulation activates the parasympathetic nervous system. In: Advances in Vibration Engineering and Structural Dynamics Francisco Beltran-Carbajal edite. Croatia: InTech; 2012. pp. 335-369. http://www.intechopen.com

[10] Hiraba H, Inoue M, Gora K, Sato T, Nishimura S, Yamaoka M, Kumakura A, Ono S, Wakasa H, Nakayama E, Abe K, Ueda K. Facial vibrotactile stimulation activates the parasympathetic nervous system: Study of salivary secretion, heart rate, pupillary reflex, and functional near-infrared spectroscopy activity. BioMed Research International. 2014;**2**:1-9

Chapter 8

Combined Approaches in Sialolithiasis of Major Salivary Glands

Iordanis Konstantinidis,
Angelos Chatziavramidis and Ioannis Iakovou

Additional information is available at the end of the chapter

http://dx.doi.org/10.5772/intechopen.72308

Abstract

Combined (endoscopic-transcutaneous/intraoral) techniques are an effective treatment for large and/or impacted stones of the major salivary glands. This approach results in high rates of symptom improvement and gland preservation. The complication rates are relatively low, further supporting the use of these techniques as an additional tool between the classic sialendoscopy and the external classic procedures of gland removal. In this chapter, we describe the combined approach for the parotid gland and the submandibular gland and finally, the retrograde sialendoscopy through the surgical field of an open approach.

Keywords: sialendoscopy, transcutaneous, sialolithiasis, parotid, submandibular

1. Introduction

Endoscopic techniques in the management of sialolithiasis were introduced since the 1990s and gradually became the standard treatment option, decreasing the external procedures [1]. In our days only 20–25% of all symptomatic cases require an open surgical approach of the gland [1, 2]. The introduction of interventional sialendoscopy with intraductal laser fragmentation did not solve all the problems as some stones were too large to be fragmented, and some others had associated with ductal stenosis which could not be dilated [3].

In order to avoid gland removal with its associated significant morbidity, surgeons developed combined techniques (endoscopic and transcutaneous) as a solution within the frame of a gland-preserving strategy [4–6].

Indications for this combined management are failure of interventional sialendoscopy to treat impacted calculi, stones larger than 8 mm, stones located behind a stenosis which cannot be dilated, and finally a non-successful extra- or intracorporeal lithotripsy [4–8].

In this chapter, we present approaches that we use in parotid and submandibular sialolithiasis cases in order to avoid gland removal.

2. Combined approach in parotid sialolithiasis

2.1. Surgical technique

This is a procedure performed under general anesthesia. Facial nerve monitoring is mandatory as in the majority of the cases a branch of the nerve is located closely to the main ductal system.

Before the procedure, a diagnostic sialendoscopy is carried out to ensure that endoscopic localization of the stone is possible. The sialendoscope used in surgery has usually a diameter of 1.1 mm. The first step of the procedure is the identification by means of the endoscope of the stone's location in the ductal system. Then, the skin above the stone is marked as the light of the endoscope's tip can be easily detected (**Figure 1**).

The location of the stone (proximal-distal, superficial-deep in the gland) is the factor which affects the surgeon's decision regarding the incision which is required. Three incisions have been described [8]:

1. Lazy S
2. Mini parotidectomy incision extended if required to face lift
3. Straight, small incision above the stone

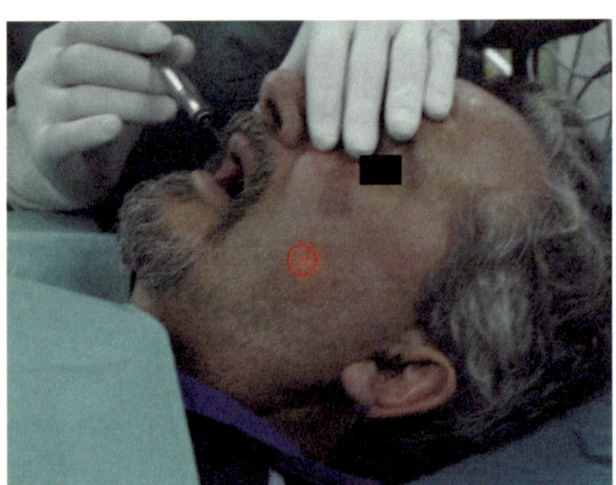

Figure 1. Transillumination of the parotid area and skin marking before the operation.

In the vast majority of cases, the first two incisions are used with the last one only in very superficial and/or proximal stones especially in aged people where the skin lines can hide a relatively small facial scar.

In cases where a parotid incision approach is required, the skin flap is elevated exposing enough surface of the gland for the stone removal. Transillumination of the sialendoscope's tip into the ductal system helps the precise gland-preserving dissection technique. In superficial stones, a longitudinal incision of the gland parenchyma (1–1.5 cm in length) above the endoscope light is performed (**Figure 2A**). In stones with deeper location (5 mm from the surface of the gland), a mini-flap of the gland parenchyma is prepared above the area of the ductal system which is lighted (**Figure 2B**) [9].

Stenting the ductal system is not obligatory. We suggest the use of a stent in cases where an opening of the ductal system larger than 1 cm has been performed and/or other traumatic manipulations in the duct have been done during removal of a polyp or an impacted stone. Usually, when a stent is used, this is placed in a retrograde fashion via the surgical field and secured in buccal mucosa with absorbable sutures (**Figure 3**). The stent can be left for a period of 3–6 weeks. The closure of the parotid duct is carried out using absorbable sutures. Fibrin glue and absorbable sutures are used for the repositioning of the gland flap in cases of non-superficial stone location (**Figure 4A** and **B**). A small drainage usually is needed as in parotid tumor surgery which is removed on the first postoperative day. Tight bandage for 4–5 days is proposed to avoid leak of saliva. Patients take broad-spectrum antibiotic treatment for a week and analgesics if required.

2.2. Follow-up assessment

During the first postoperative period (2–3 weeks), patients are advised to avoid nutrition which produce excessive saliva (e.g., lemon juice, etc.).

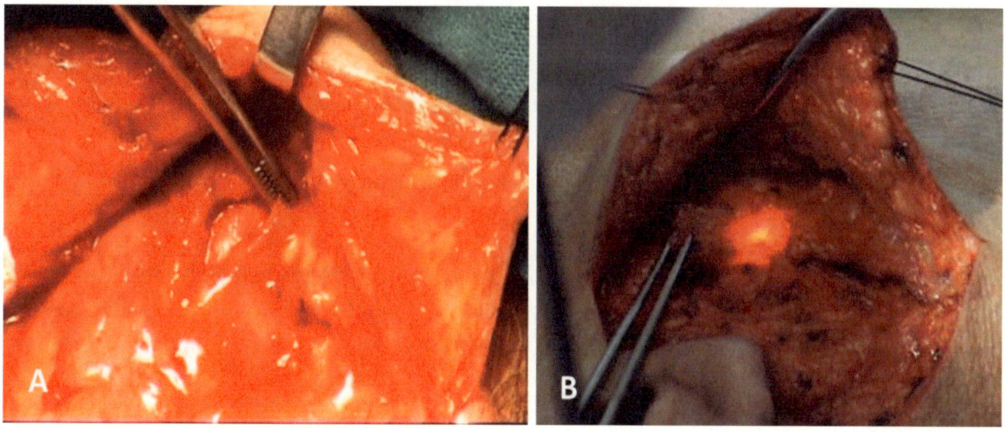

Figure 2. (A) Longitudinal incision of the gland in a superficial stone and (B) ⊓-shaped mini-flap in a deep-located stone.

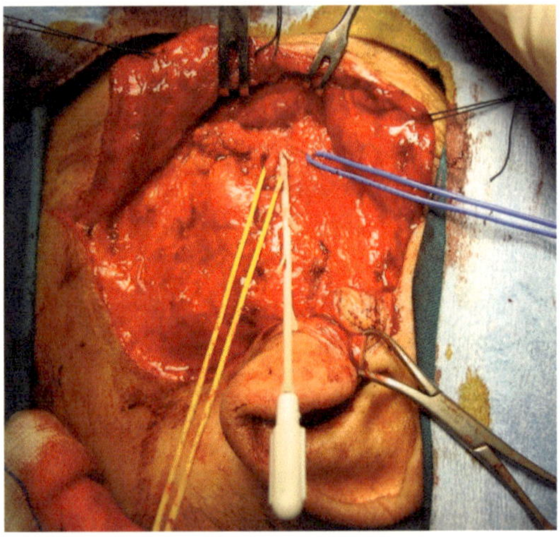

Figure 3. Stent placement in a retrograde fashion via the surgical field. The left loop isolates the main duct, and the right the facial nerve branch which run close to the ductal system.

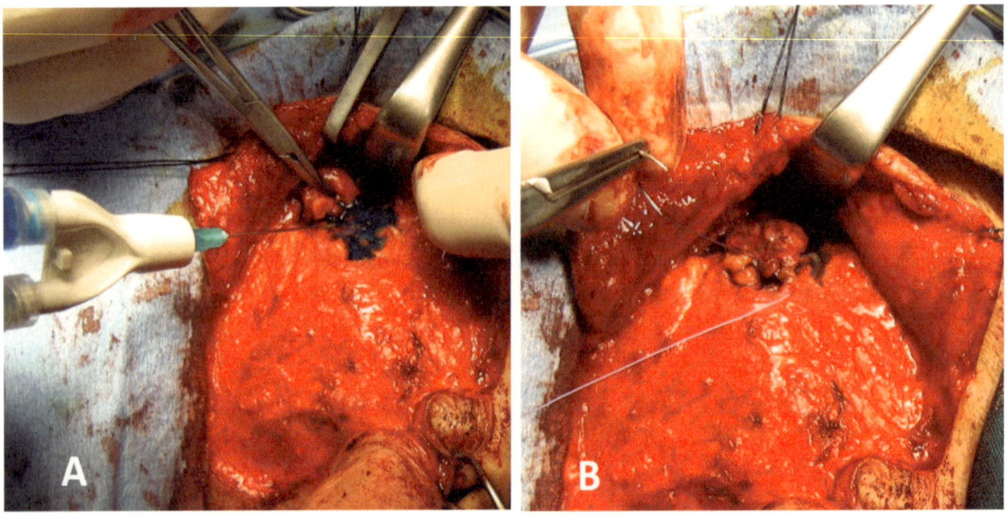

Figure 4. (A) Fibrin glue and (B) absorbable sutures are used for the repositioning of the gland flap in cases of non-superficial stone location.

Early complications such as hematoma, sialadenitis, wound infection, fistula, and obstructed and/or extruded stent have been rarely published and usually occur within the first postoperative month. In such cases, conservative management and removal of stent if needed are enough measures [9–11].

Initially, one of the surgeons' concerns about the procedure was the potential postoperative stenosis at the site of the ductal incision. This fact is expected and was confirmed in our data, as 7 patients out of 12 had an endoscopically diagnosed postoperative stenosis [9]. However, these stenotic areas are considered without clinical impact as none of the patients suffered from postoperative swellings. The incision is parallel to the duct axon, and this may decrease the possibility for severe stenosis even in cases with extended opening. In addition stenting with precise intraoperative placement can be helpful to avoid postoperative stenosis. Undoubtedly, further studies are needed to justify the size of the ductal opening which is critical regarding postoperative stenosis.

In the same study, scintigraphic evaluation of the operated parotid glands in two phases (baseline and after stimulation) provided an objective functional evaluation 1 year after the procedures [9]. Specifically, a dynamic imaging of the whole anterior head started after a bolus intravenous injection of ^{99m}Tc. Fifteen minutes after the initial injection, diluted lemon juice was given per oz. The parameters measured were (1) uptake rate, taken as the value of the initial slope of the time-activity curve and (2) washout fraction, as a relative mobilized radioactivity from each parotid gland after the sialogogue's application. In the vast majority of cases (11/12), the procedure preserved the function of the gland with only one parotid hypofunction in a patient with long-term history of sialolithiasis.

Extracorporeal and laser intraductal lithotripsy requires expensive devices which are not always available; they are time-consuming and always have a potential risk of leaving residual stone fragments which can be a nidus for new stone formation. Moreover, some patients prefer the described surgical option as a "one shoot" intervention instead of extracorporeal lithotripsy which may need multiple sessions [10–12].

Contraindication for this procedure is the presence of diffuse ductal stenosis or multiple parenchymal stones [8, 9].

3. Combined approach in submandibular sialolithiasis

A combined approach can be also used for submandibular gland with large and/or impacted stones in a similar manner with the parotid gland.

3.1. Surgical technique

The procedure starts again with a sialendoscopy, and when the endoscope approximates, the stone then is fixed to the floor of the mouth or can be held steadily by an assistant.

Infiltration of the transilluminated area with xylocaine 2%-adrenalin 1% solution follows. The next step is an incision of the oral mucosa approximately 2 cm in length following the axis of Wharton's duct size just above the lighted area (**Figure 5A** and **B**). Caution should be taken at this point in order to avoid lingual nerve damage as it crosses Wharton's duct and this is the reason why some authors identify and isolate the nerve with a loop from the surgical field [8].

A useful surgical tip is the fact that the floor of the mouth can be pushed upward by external pressure at submandibular triangle below the patient's mandible, giving better access to the hilum area endorally.

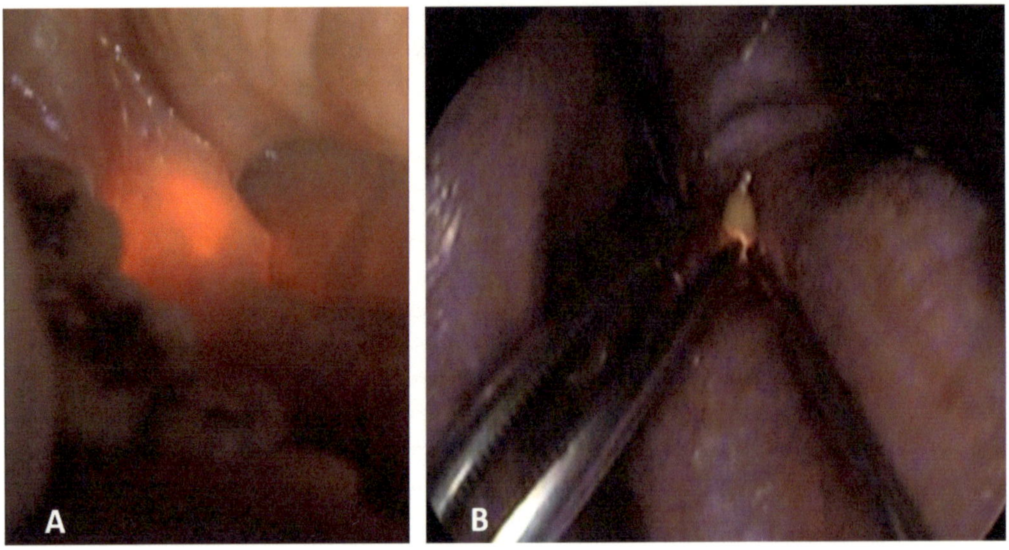

Figure 5. (A) Transillumination of the hilum area in a right submandibular gland intaraorally. (B) Incision and stone removal.

After the identification of the duct, silastic loops are positioned around the duct helping its traction and dissection. The stone is palpated by the finger or surgical instrument, and a straight incision above the stone at the axis of the duct is performed. Once the stone has been removed, an endoscopy of the ductal system behind the stone is mandatory for residual stones or strictures, etc.

The use of a stent at the end of the procedure is not universally accepted; however, it is the preference of the authors as it offers a stable floor for the ductoplasty. Its insertion through the papilla can be performed directly or with the use of the endoscope or a guide-wire for more safety especially when a precise placement to the posterior portion of the duct is required. The stent is then sutured and secured with a nonabsorbable suture to Wharton's papilla area. The time of stenting varies in the literature with a period of 3 weeks being the minimum and 6 weeks usually the maximum depending on the patients' tolerance.

3.2. Follow-up assessment

Patients receive the same instructions as in parotid stones for their diet postoperatively. Similarly, they take broad-spectrum antibiotic treatment for a week and analgesics if required with the addition of oral antiseptic solution local application after meals.

Early complications are rare and include lingual nerve damage, hematoma, and gland swelling extrusion of the stent which are usually managed in a conservative way.

A certain degree of postoperative stenosis is expected in the long term; however, the region of the hilum is large enough, and these strictures run usually as asymptomatic.

This procedure is not popular in the literature as the parotid one, because many surgeons prefer the endoral marsipulization of the duct to have access in stones at the region of the hilum. This procedure offers equally good results although does not preserve the integrity of the ductal system. Moreover, when marsipulization of the main duct reaches the hilum, the endoscopic assessment of the residual ductal system becomes problematic due to leakage during saline irrigation.

4. Retrograde sialendoscopy

In cases with parenchymal and especially multiple stones of the submandibular gland, an external approach with removal of the gland is indicated. However, some stones may slip into Wharton's duct during surgical manipulations causing symptoms at a later time. In a study by Milton et al., authors found that 5% of patients who underwent submandibular gland removal had residual stones in the remaining duct, requiring further surgery [13].

For such cases a retrograde sialendoscopy is proposed through the surgical field after the removal of the gland [14]. A standard procedure of submandibular gland resection is performed with a transcervical incision. Identification and preservation of the lingual nerve from the gland at the area of submandibular ganglion follow along with careful dissection and skeletonization of the submandibular duct. Two stay sutures are placed on the opposing sides of the duct, proximal to the gland. After the removal of the gland, these sutures are used for stretching of the duct in order to facilitate placement of a large in outer diameter (1.4 or 1.6 mm) sialendoscope for retrograde inspection (**Figure 6**).

In cases where residual stones or debris are identified, then they can be removed by wire basket or alternatively can be pushed by the endoscope into the oral cavity (retrograde) or into the neck with the endoscope coming from the oral cavity. At the end of the procedure, stay sutures help for duct traction into the neck and its ligation proximally in order to minimize the length of the remained duct.

Contraindication of this procedure is the diffuse stenosis of the duct or severe strictures due previous trauma or surgery.

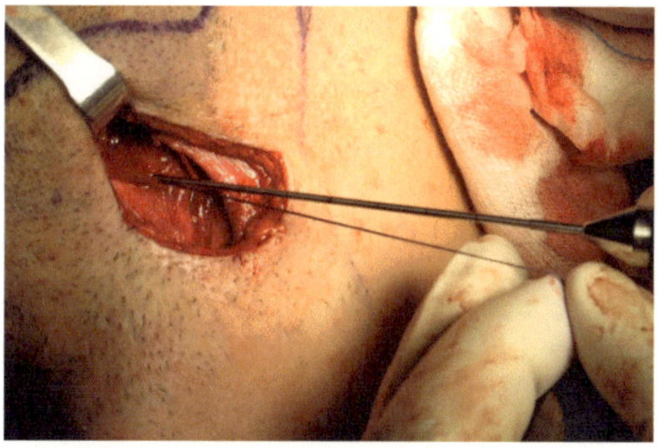

Figure 6. Retrograde sialendoscopy: insertion of the sialendoscope into Wharton's duct after removal of the submandibular gland. The duct is stretched with a silk suture.

Author details

Iordanis Konstantinidis[1]*, Angelos Chatziavramidis[1] and Ioannis Iakovou[2]

*Address all correspondence to: jordan_orl@hotmail.com

1 2nd Academic ORL Department, Aristotle University, Papageorgiou Hospital, Thessaloniki, Greece

2 3rd Nuclear Medicine Department, Aristotle University, Papageorgiou Hospital, Thessaloniki, Greece

References

[1] Iro H, Zenk J, Escudier MP, Nahlieli O, Capaccio P, Katz P, Brown J, McGurk M. Outcome of minimally invasive management of salivary calculi in 4,691 patients. The Laryngoscope. 2009;**119**:263-268. DOI: 10.1002/lary.20008

[2] Koch M, Zenk J, Iro H. Algorithms for treatment of salivary gland obstructions. Otolaryngologic Clinics of North America. 2009;**42**:1173-1192. DOI: 10.1016/j.otc.2009.08.002

[3] Phillips J, Withrow K. Outcomes of holmium laser-assisted lithotripsy with sialendoscopy in treatment of sialolithiasis. Otolaryngology and Head and Neck Surgery. 2014;**150**: 962-967. DOI: 10.1177/0194599814524716

[4] McGurk M, MacBean AD, Fan KF, Sproat C, Darwish C. Endoscopically assisted operative retrieval of parotid stones. The British Journal of Oral & Maxillofacial Surgery. 2006;**44**:157-160. DOI: 10.1016/j.bjoms.2005.03.026

[5] Walvekar RR, Bomeli SR, Carrau RL, Schaitkin B. Combined approach technique for the management ofl arge salivary stones. The Laryngoscope. 2009;**119**:1125-1129. DOI: 10.1002/lary.20203

[6] Koch M, Iro H, Zenk J. Combined endoscopic-transcutaneous surgery in parotid gland sialolithiasis and other ductal diseases: Reporting medium- to long-term objective and patients' subjective outcomes. European Archives of Oto-Rhino-Laryngology. 2013;**270**: 1933-1940. DOI: 10.1007/s00405-012-2286-y

[7] Roland LT, Skillington SA, Ogden MA. Sialendoscopy-assisted transfacial removal of parotid sialoliths: A systematic review and meta-analysis. The Laryngoscope. DOI: 10.1002/lary.26610

[8] Marchal F. A combined endoscopic and external approach for extraction of large stones with preservation of parotid and submandibular glands. The Laryngoscope. 2007;**117**: 373-377. DOI: 10.1097/mlg.0b013e31802c06e9

[9] Konstantinidis I, Chatziavramidis A, Iakovou I, Constantinidis J. Long-term results of combined approach in parotid sialolithiasis. European Archives of Oto-Rhino-Laryngology. 2015;**272**:3533-3538. DOI: 10.1007/s00405-014-3391-x

[10] Kopec T, Szyfter W, Wierzbicka M. Sialoendoscopy and combined approach for the management of salivary gland stones. European Archives of Oto-Rhino-Laryngology. 2013;**270**: 219-223. DOI: 10.1007/s00405-012-2145-x

[11] Klein H, Ardekian L. The treatment of large sialoliths by sialendoscopic combined approach. Journal of Oral and Maxillofacial Surgery. 2014;**72**:737-743. DOI: 10.1016/j.joms.2013.09.003

[12] Capaccio P, Torretta S, Pignataro L, Koch M. Salivary lithotripsy in the era of sialendoscopy. Acta Otorhinolaryngologica Italica. 2017;**37**:113-121. DOI: 10.14639/0392-100X-1600

[13] Milton CM, Thomas BM, Bickerton RC. Morbidity study of submandibular gland excision. Annals of the Royal College of Surgeons of England. 1986;**68**:148-150

[14] Potash A, Hoffman HT. Retrograde sialendoscopy: A new technique for avoiding retained ductal stones. The Annals of Otology, Rhinology, and Laryngology. 2012;**121**:38-43. DOI: 10.1177/000348941212100107